This Journal Belongs to:

____

If lost, please contact:

____

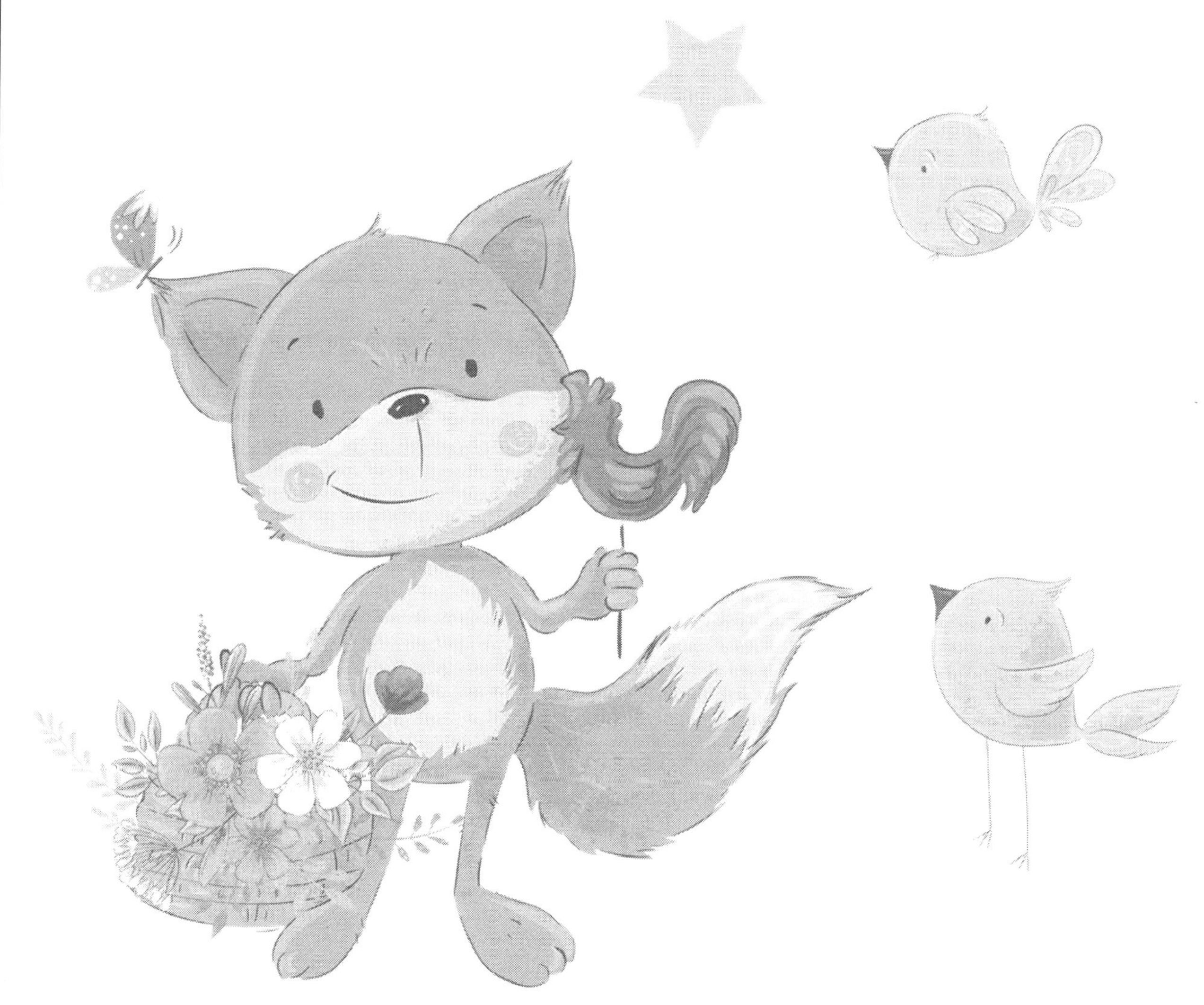

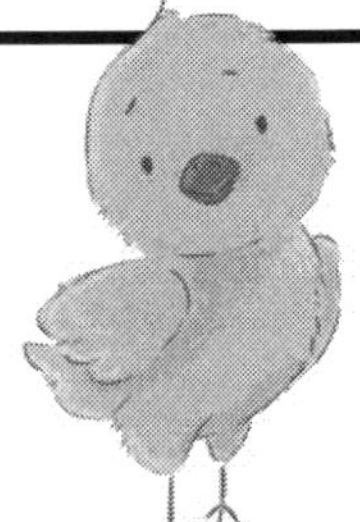

You're expecting! Here's what you can expect in this Pregnancy Journal:

NEW & IMPROVED pages to enjoy your pregnancy! Here is what's included in this journal:

- Pregnancy Journal Pages to record memorable events for Weeks 4 – 41 (just in case you're overdue!) AND to include a weekly photo of the baby bump or an alternate photo/drawing that you prefer or to tell your growing baby something you want him/her to know. Fun Facts are included about baby's growth every week.
- Additional blank pages to freely journal whatever you want.
- 3 journal pages to summarize each of your trimesters
- Fun Predictions About Baby's Birth
- Space for both moms to write "My First Love Letter to My Baby"
- Space for listing your Baby Name Ideas
- Growing a Healthy Baby Meal Planner
- Foods/Drinks to Avoid & Ones to Add to Your Shopping List
- Exercise During Pregnancy – Questions that Need Answering
- Newborn Baby Shopping List
- Maternity Hospital Bag Checklist
- Record of Prenatal Appointments
- Our Baby Shower
- Our Sonogram Photos or space to describe the ultrasound(s)
- Fetal Movements Tracking Charts
- Our Birth Plan
- Our Nursery Room Ideas
- Our Family Tree (includes both Mommies)
- Important Pre-Birth Questions & Considerations
- The Birth and space for First Family Photos

About Your Parents

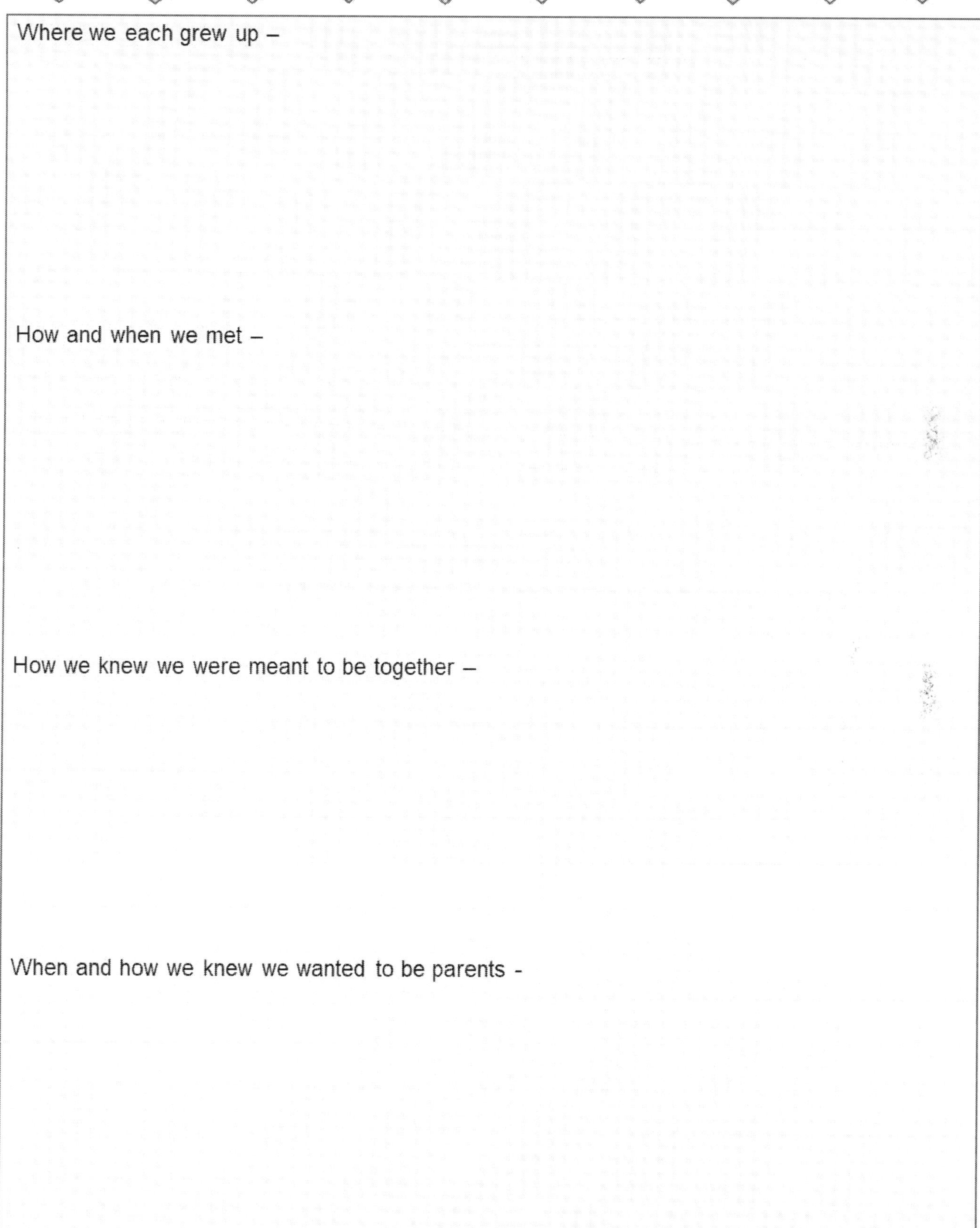

We Are Trying to Conceive

Our journey of conception:

How long it took to get pregnant:

A photo, drawing, or a story of your mom and mom before you were born:

We Are Pregnant!

Our Estimated Due Date:

Date we found out:

How far along were we?:

How we found out:

Our reactions:

Did we suspect we were pregnant?:

Who we first told about the pregnancy & their reactions:

What else do we remember about the day we found out that we were expecting?:

Before You Were Born

Prices of Common Items

Loaf of bread:

Can of soda/pop:

A dozen eggs:

Chocolate bar:

Gallon of milk:

Toothpaste:

Body wash:

Antiperspirant:

Average home purchase:

______________:

Arts & Culture

Popular movies of the year:

Popular songs of the year:

Price of a movie:

World Events

President/Prime Minister of our country:

Notable world events going on:

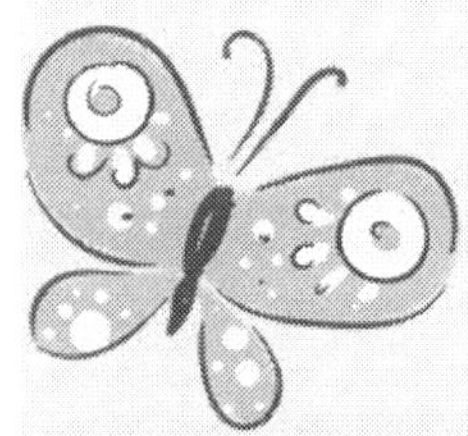

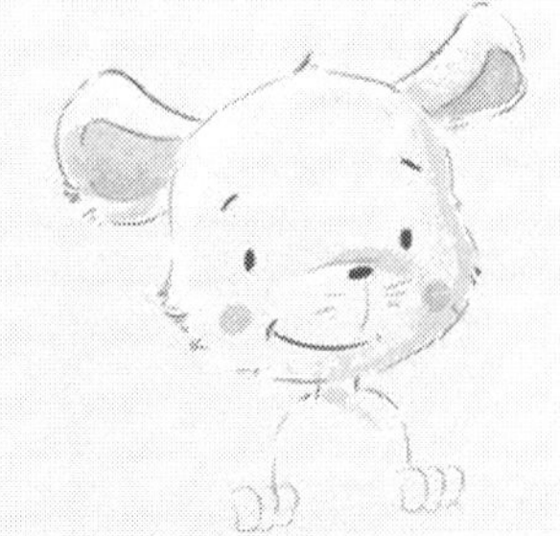

Our Pregnancy Journal

Week 4

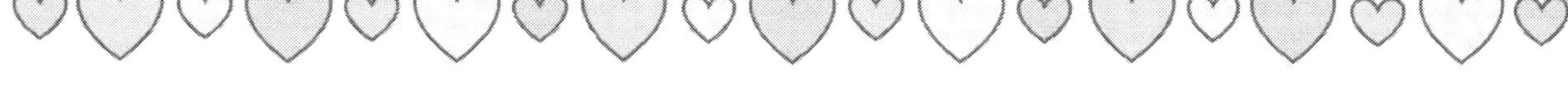

Baby Bump

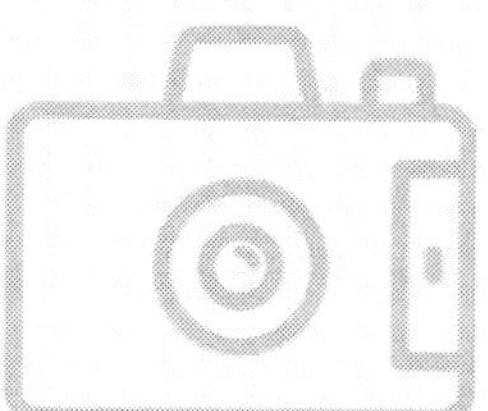

Compare the size of your growing baby throughout the pregnancy by remembering to take a photo and then adding it in this location on each page every week OR, if you prefer, use this space to write about how you're both feeling or things you want to tell your growing baby.

My Weight:

Belly Circumference:

Baby in Progress....Fun Facts

* Baby is the size of a poppy seed.

* Your baby is a ball of cells that are rapidly multiplying.

* The primitive placenta is developing.

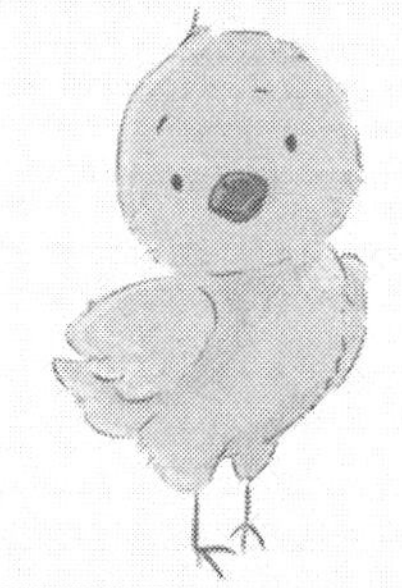

What we want to remember most about this week:

Our Pregnancy Journal

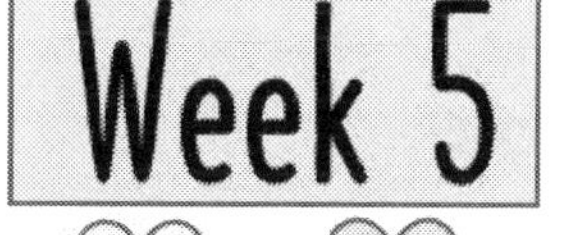

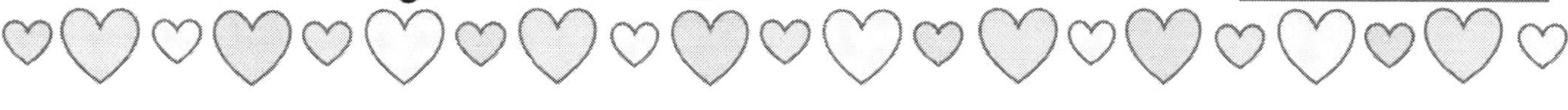

Baby Bump

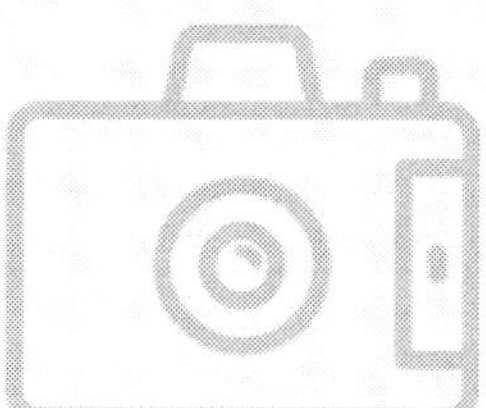

Compare the size of your growing baby throughout the pregnancy by remembering to take a photo and then adding it in this location on each page every week OR, if you prefer, use this space to write about how you're both feeling or things you want to tell your growing baby.

My Weight:

Belly Circumference:

Baby in Progress....Fun Facts

* Baby is the size of a sesame seed.
* The neural tube, which eventually forms the brain and spinal cord is developing.
* The heart is developing too.
* Mom may be feeling tired and nauseous as her body works hard to create this new life.

What we want to remember most about this week:

Our Pregnancy Journal

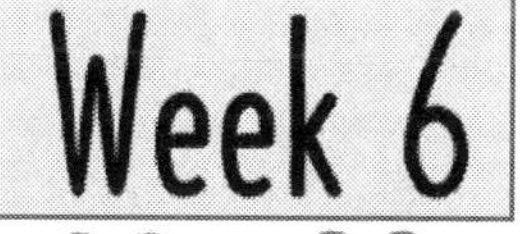

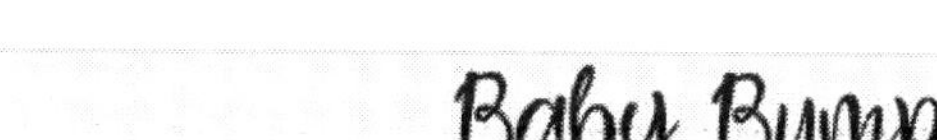

Baby Bump

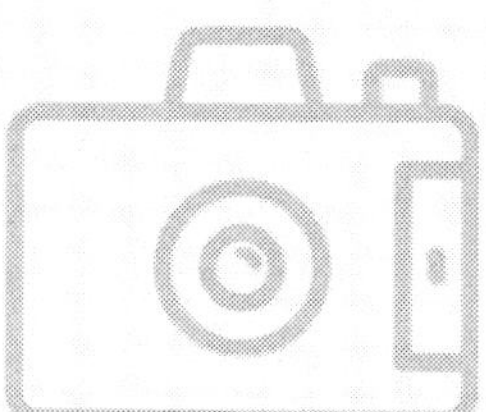

Compare the size of your growing baby throughout the pregnancy by remembering to take a photo and then adding it in this location on each page every week OR, if you prefer, use this space to write about how you're both feeling or things you want to tell your growing baby.

My Weight:

Belly Circumference:

Baby in Progress....Fun Facts

* Baby is the size of a lentil or pomegranate seed, approx. ¼".
* The neural tube in baby's back closes, heart & other organs (lungs) are developing, small arm buds appear, & eyes & ears primitively form.
* Baby's heart starts to beat!

What we want to remember most about this week:

Our Pregnancy Journal

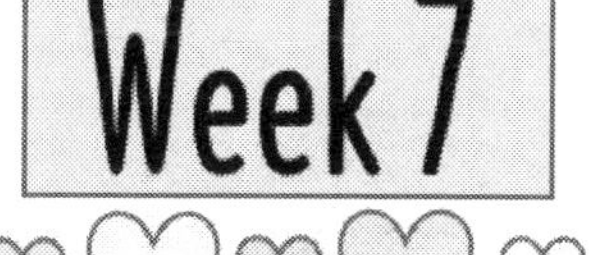

Baby Bump

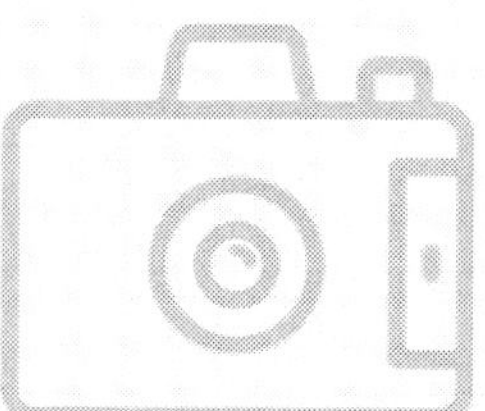

Compare the size of your growing baby throughout the pregnancy by remembering to take a photo and then adding it in this location on each page every week OR, if you prefer, use this space to write about how you're both feeling or things you want to tell your growing baby.

My Weight:

Belly Circumference:

Baby in Progress....Fun Facts

* Baby has doubled in size since last week, and is now the size of a blueberry.
* Baby's brain & head are growing, nostrils and retinas are starting to develop, leg buds appear, & the arm buds now look like paddles.
* The placenta burrows into the wall of the uterus.

What we want to remember most about this week:

Our Pregnancy Journal

Week 8

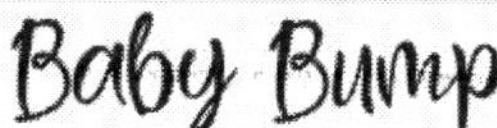

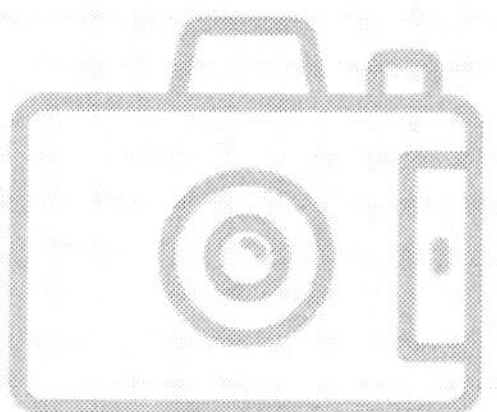

My Weight:

Belly Circumference:

Baby in Progress....Fun Facts

* Baby is the size of a kidney bean or a raspberry, and over ½" long from head to rump.
* Fingers and nose are forming, and the leg buds look like paddles.
* Although you cannot feel it yet, baby moves a lot.

What we want to remember most about this week:

Our Pregnancy Journal

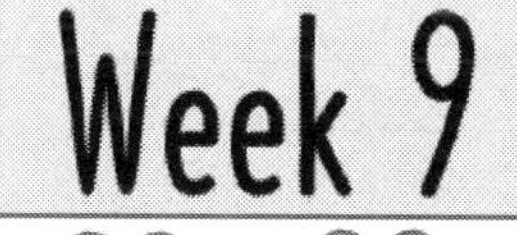

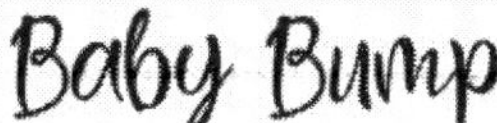

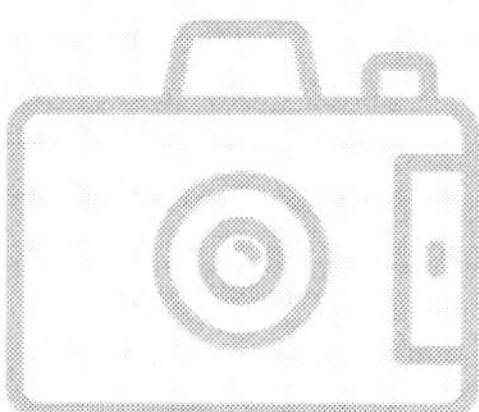

My Weight:

Belly Circumference:

Baby in Progress....Fun Facts

* Baby is roughly the size of a grape or a cherry.
* The eyes are fully formed, but closed.
* Baby's eyelids form, baby's arms grow, elbows appear, & toes are developing.
* The reproductive organs are forming, but you cannot tell if it's a boy or girl yet.

What we want to remember most about this week:

Our Pregnancy Journal

Week 10

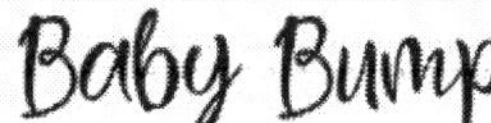

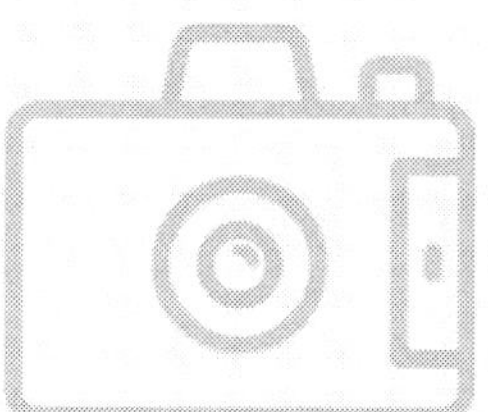

My Weight:

Belly Circumference:

Baby in Progress....Fun Facts

* Baby is the size of a kumquat, measures a bit over 1" from head to buttocks.
* All of the baby's organs are now formed.
* Baby's brain is active with brain waves!
* Baby can bend the elbows, and the toes & fingers are no longer webbed in appearance as they get longer, and the head gets rounder.

What we want to remember most about this week:

Our Pregnancy Journal

Week 11

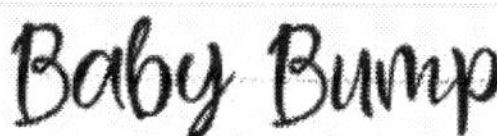

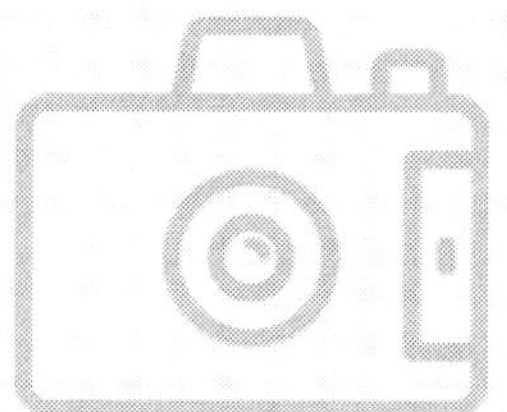

My Weight:

Belly Circumference:

Baby in Progress....Fun Facts

* Baby is the size of a fig, over 1.5" long from the top of the head to the buttocks, & can kick & stretch.
* Early teeth buds are developing in the mouth.
* Baby's fingernails are also growing, but are not full length for several weeks.
* Baby's head is large and makes up more than half of baby's length at this time.

What we want to remember most about this week:

Our Pregnancy Journal

Week 12

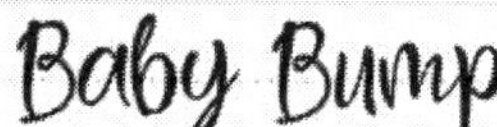

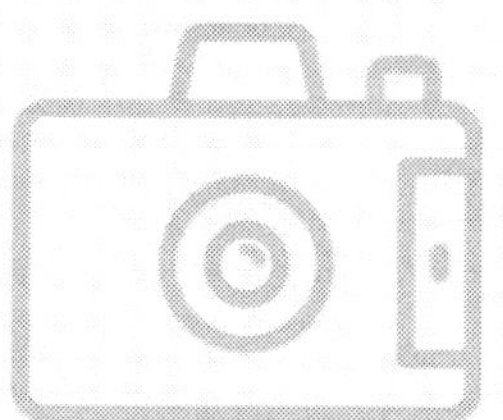

My Weight:

Belly Circumference:

Baby in Progress....Fun Facts

* Baby is the size of a lime or a plum, and is over 2" long from head to butt.
* Baby's kidneys are working, and starting to excrete urine.
* Baby's bones are developing.
* Baby is opening & closing his/her fingers, and kicking his/her arms and legs.

What we want to remember most about this week:

Our First Trimester

Weeks 1-12

What we enjoyed most & least about the first trimester

How We Felt This Trimester

Our Favorite Memories

Our Pregnancy Journal

Week 13

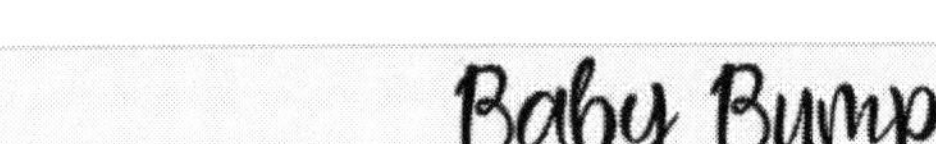

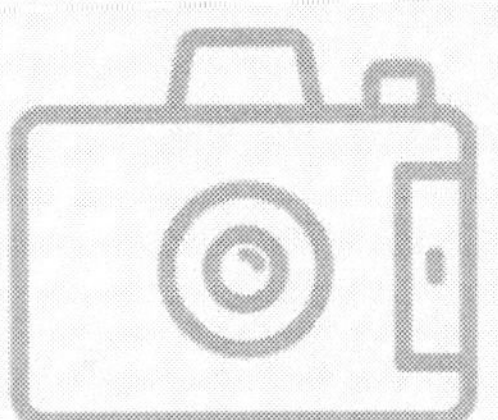

My Weight:

Belly Circumference:

Baby in Progress....Fun Facts

* Baby is the size of a pea pod, is approx. 3" long, & weighs 1 oz.
* Your baby's vocal cords & fingerprints are forming.
* The baby bump may be noticeable to family & friends.
* Your baby swims in utero.
* Baby girl's ovaries are filled with eggs for future procreation.
* Baby's head only makes up about 1/3 of the baby's length now.

What we want to remember most about this week:

Our Pregnancy Journal

Week 14

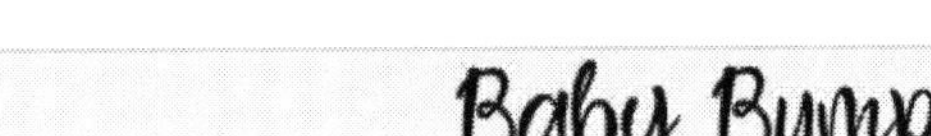

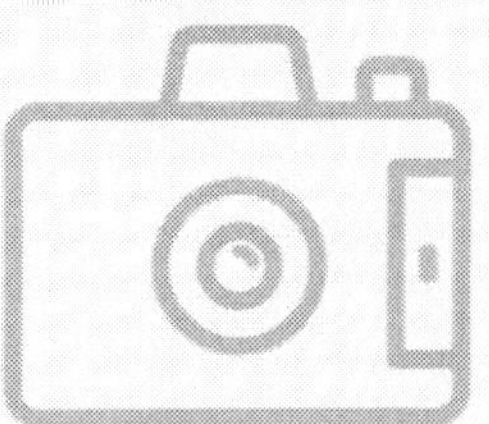

My Weight:

Belly Circumference:

Baby in Progress....Fun Facts

*Baby is the size of a lemon or small peach, 3.5" long, & can make some facial expressions.

* Baby exhibits sucking reflexes. He/she is also growing fine-like hair (lanugo) on his/her body, but most or all of it will disappear before birth of full-term babies.

* All of baby's internal organs are now formed, and will mature as baby grows in the uterus over the coming months.

What we want to remember most about this week:

Our Pregnancy Journal

Week 15

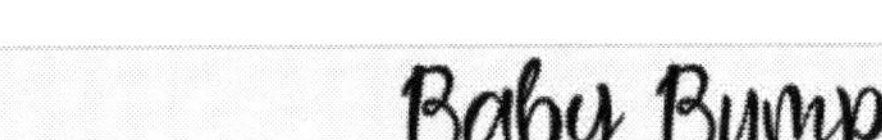

Baby Bump

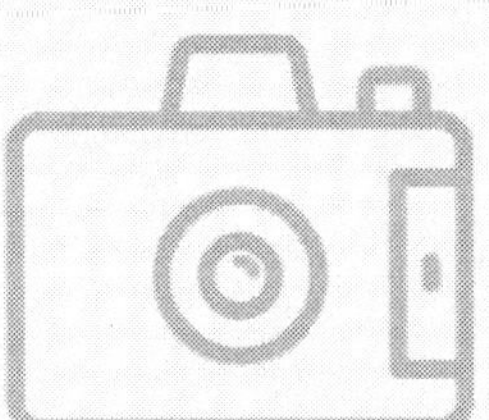

My Weight:

Belly Circumference:

Baby in Progress....Fun Facts

* Baby is the size of an apple, 4" long, & 2.5 oz.
* Baby's muscles are getting stronger, so baby is using them to make fists and perform somersaults in utero. There is still a lot of space in the womb.
* Baby's closed eyes are starting to be sensitive to light.
* Baby may suck his/her thumb.
* Taste buds are starting to develop.

What we want to remember most about this week:

Our Pregnancy Journal

Week 16

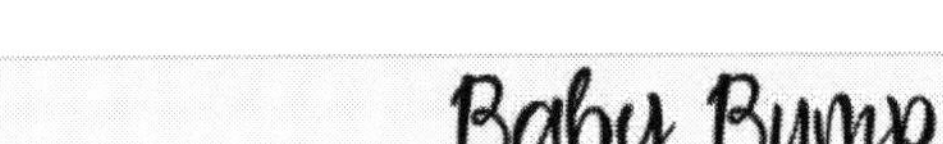

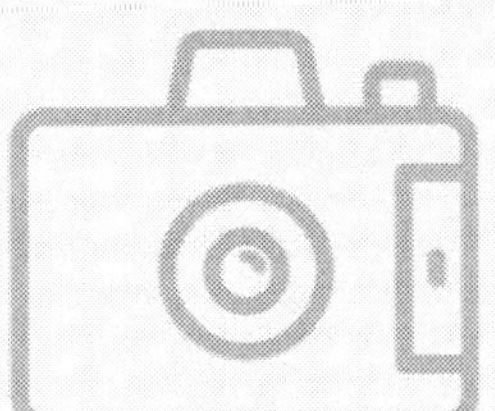

My Weight:

Belly Circumference:

Baby in Progress....Fun Facts

* Baby is the size of an avocado, over 4.5" long from top of the head to buttocks, and roughly 3.5 oz.
* Baby's heart is pumping around 49 pints (28 L) of blood around his/her body every day!
* Eyebrows and eyelashes are forming.
* Fine hair (lanugo) is still growing on the baby's body to help regulate temperature and protect it from the amniotic fluid.

What we want to remember most about this week:

Our Pregnancy Journal

Week 17

Baby Bump

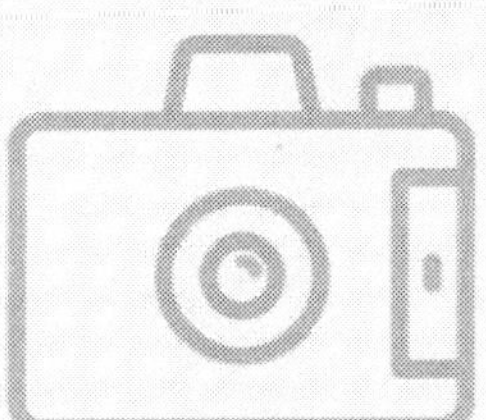

My Weight:

Belly Circumference:

Baby in Progress....Fun Facts

* Baby is roughly the size of a turnip, weighs 5 oz, & is 5" long.
* Baby's hearing is pretty good, & can hear your muffled voice & music.
* Baby's head of hair is growing.
* Baby's lungs practice by breathing in amniotic fluid in the womb.

What we want to remember most about this week:

Our Pregnancy Journal

Week 18

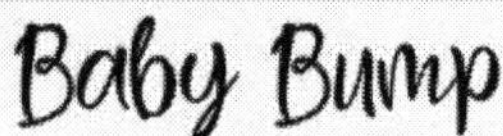

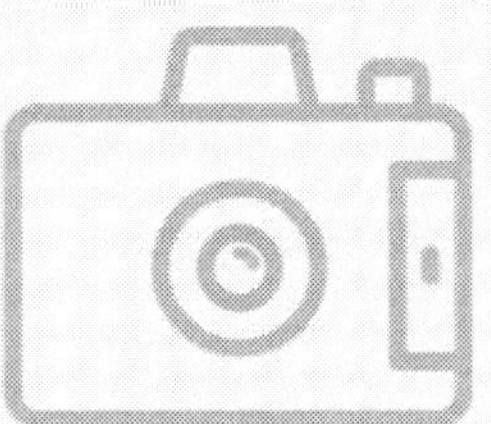

My Weight:

Belly Circumference:

Baby in Progress....Fun Facts

* Baby is the size of a bell pepper, weighs 7 oz, & is 5.5" long from head to buttocks.
* Any day, baby's movements may be felt from within the womb.
* An ultrasound now can identify if you're having a girl or boy.
* Be sure to talk and sing to baby as his/her ears can hear you.

What we want to remember most about this week:

Our Pregnancy Journal

Week 19

Baby Bump

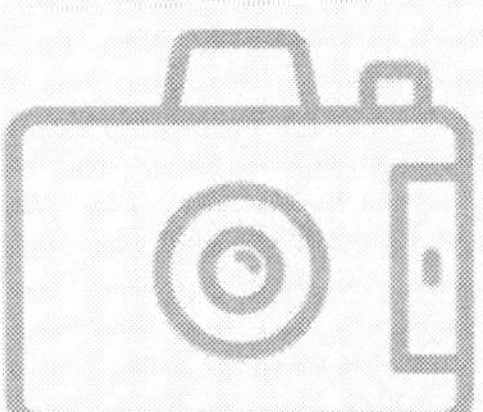

My Weight:

Belly Circumference:

Baby in Progress....Fun Facts

* Baby is the size of a mango, weighs 8.5 oz, & is 6" long.
* Baby's skin is covered with a waxy substance called vernix caseosa, which also protects it from the amniotic fluid.
* Baby is starting to put on early fat, which is important for temperature control when born.

What we want to remember most about this week:

Our Pregnancy Journal

Week 20

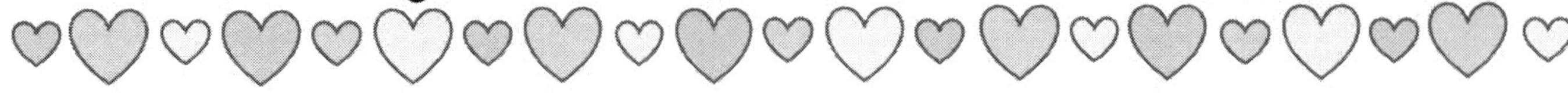

Baby Bump

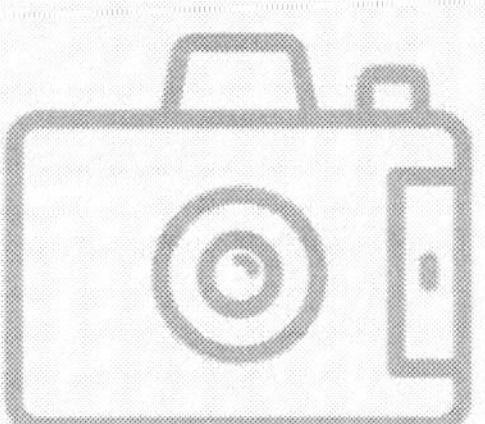

My Weight:

Belly Circumference:

Baby in Progress....Fun Facts

* It's the halfway point in the pregnancy!
* Baby is the size of a banana, & is 6.5" from head to butt or 10" to the heels.
* Your baby is going to continue to grow, and so will the belly.

What we want to remember most about this week:

Our Pregnancy Journal

Week 21

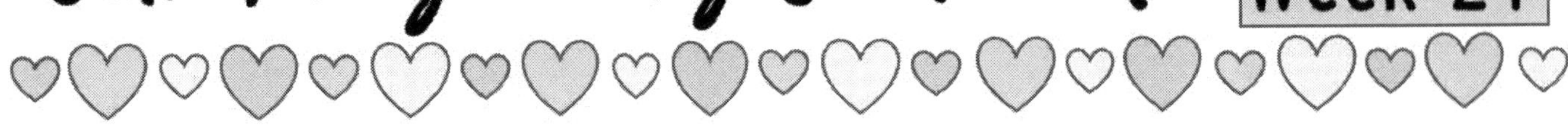

Baby Bump

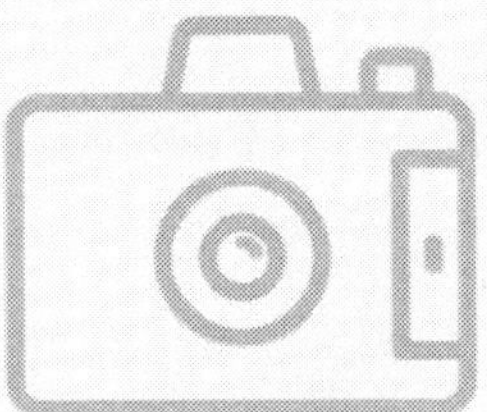

My Weight:

Belly Circumference:

Baby in Progress....Fun Facts

* Baby is 10.5" long (like a carrot), & weighs approximately 12 oz.
* Baby's eyes move rapidly under the eyelids.
* Baby's intestines and bowels are starting to produce meconium, which will be baby's first poo after birth.

What we want to remember most about this week:

Our Pregnancy Journal

Week 22

Baby Bump

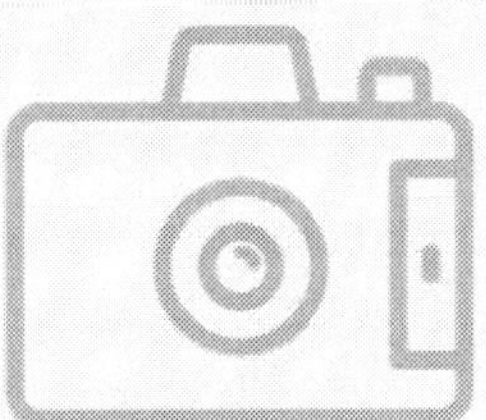

My Weight:

Belly Circumference:

Baby in Progress….Fun Facts

* Baby is the size of a spaghetti squash, weighs 1 lb, & is 10" to 11" long from head to butt.
* Baby's body (lungs, etc.) continues to develop and specialize in preparation for eventual birth.
* If it is a boy, the testes begin to descend into the scrotum.

What we want to remember most about this week:

Our Pregnancy Journal

Week 23

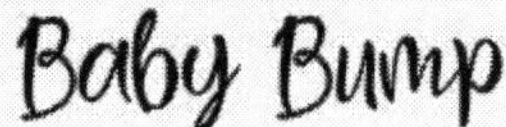

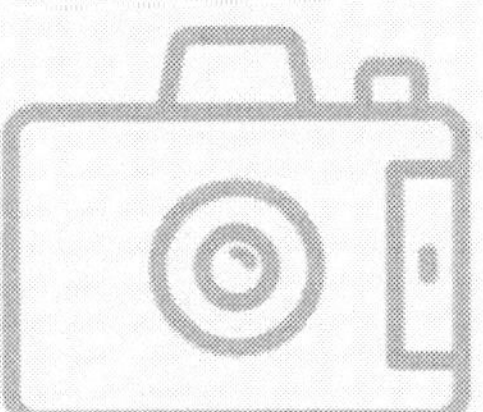

My Weight:

Belly Circumference:

Baby in Progress....Fun Facts

* Baby is the size of a grapefruit.
* Baby still has several more weeks of growing within the womb, but is practicing breathing by breathing in amniotic fluid. The lungs are also producing a surfactant product that will allow the lungs to work properly with less surface tension.
* Baby's brain continues to specialize & produce more complex links.

What we want to remember most about this week:

Our Pregnancy Journal

Week 24

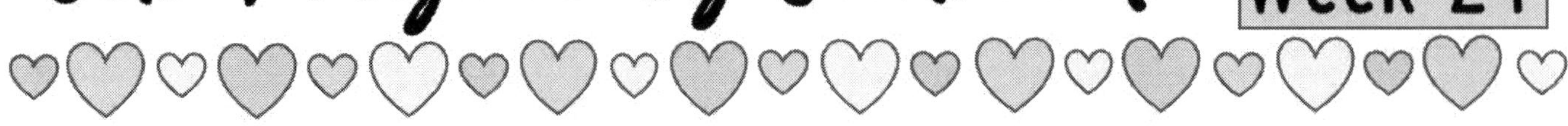

Baby Bump

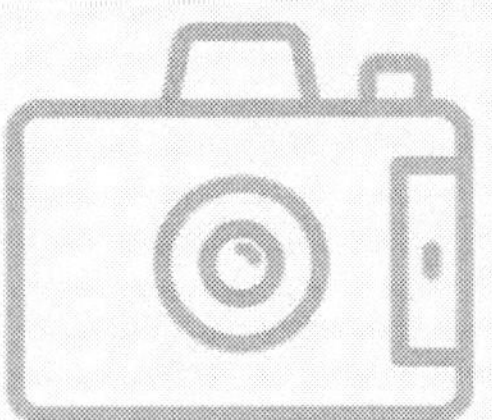

My Weight:

Belly Circumference:

Baby in Progress....Fun Facts

* Baby is about 12" (30 cm) long, & weighs 1 ¼ lb.
* Baby continues to practice breathing within the womb.
* Fat continues to develop under the skin for thermoregulation.
* Baby is considered possibly "viable" if he/she is born now, but really needs more time to grow & maximize the chances for survival outside the womb.

What we want to remember most about this week:

Our Pregnancy Journal

Week 25

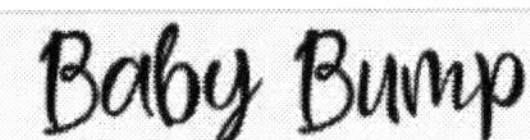

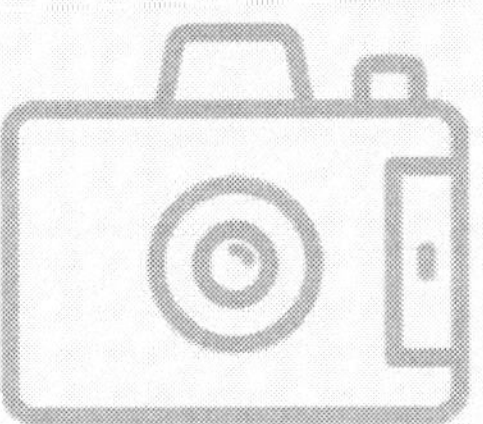

My Weight:

Belly Circumference:

Baby in Progress....Fun Facts

* Baby is the size of a rutabaga. It is about 13.5" in length, & 1 ½ lb.
* Your baby can stick his/her tongue out!
* Your baby's skin is becoming more opaque (less see-through).

What we want to remember most about this week:

Our Pregnancy Journal

Week 26

Baby Bump

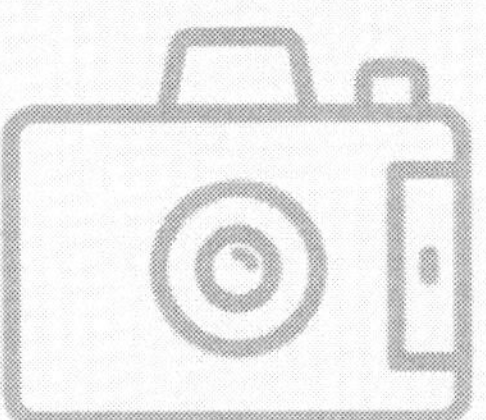

My Weight:

Belly Circumference:

Baby in Progress....Fun Facts

* Baby is 14" long, roughly the length of a zucchini, and 1 & 2/3 lb.
* Your baby's eyes are now open!
* Trying shining a light on the pregnant belly, and baby may kick back in response.

What we want to remember most about this week:

Our Pregnancy Journal

Week 27

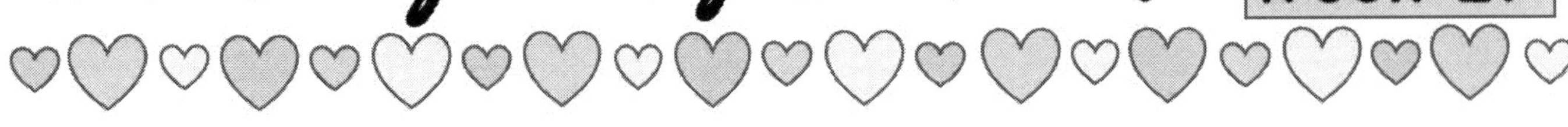

Baby Bump

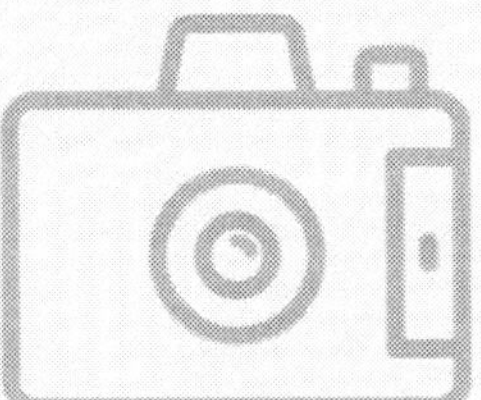

My Weight:

Belly Circumference:

Baby in Progress....Fun Facts

* Baby is the size of a cauliflower, is 14.5" long, & 2 lb in weight.
* Baby has the ability to distinguish voices outside of the womb.
* Baby has noticeable periods of wakefulness and sleeping.
* Baby's brain and organs are maturing and growing.
* Hiccups may be felt from within the womb.

What we want to remember most about this week:

Our Pregnancy Journal

Week 28

Baby Bump

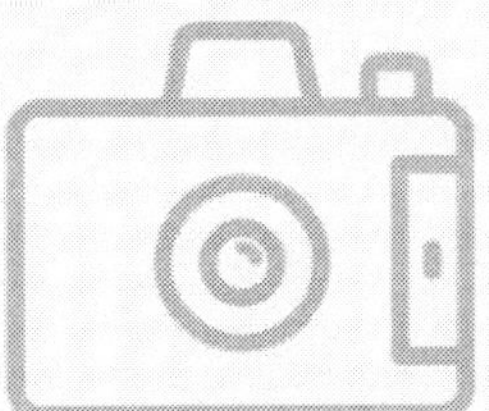

My Weight:

Belly Circumference:

Baby in Progress....Fun Facts

* Baby is the size of an eggplant, weighs 2 ¼ lb,, & is 15'' long.
* Baby's body has finally caught up with the fast growth of the head in early weeks.
* Your baby can blink his/her eyes.

What we want to remember most about this week:

Our Second Trimester

Weeks 13-28

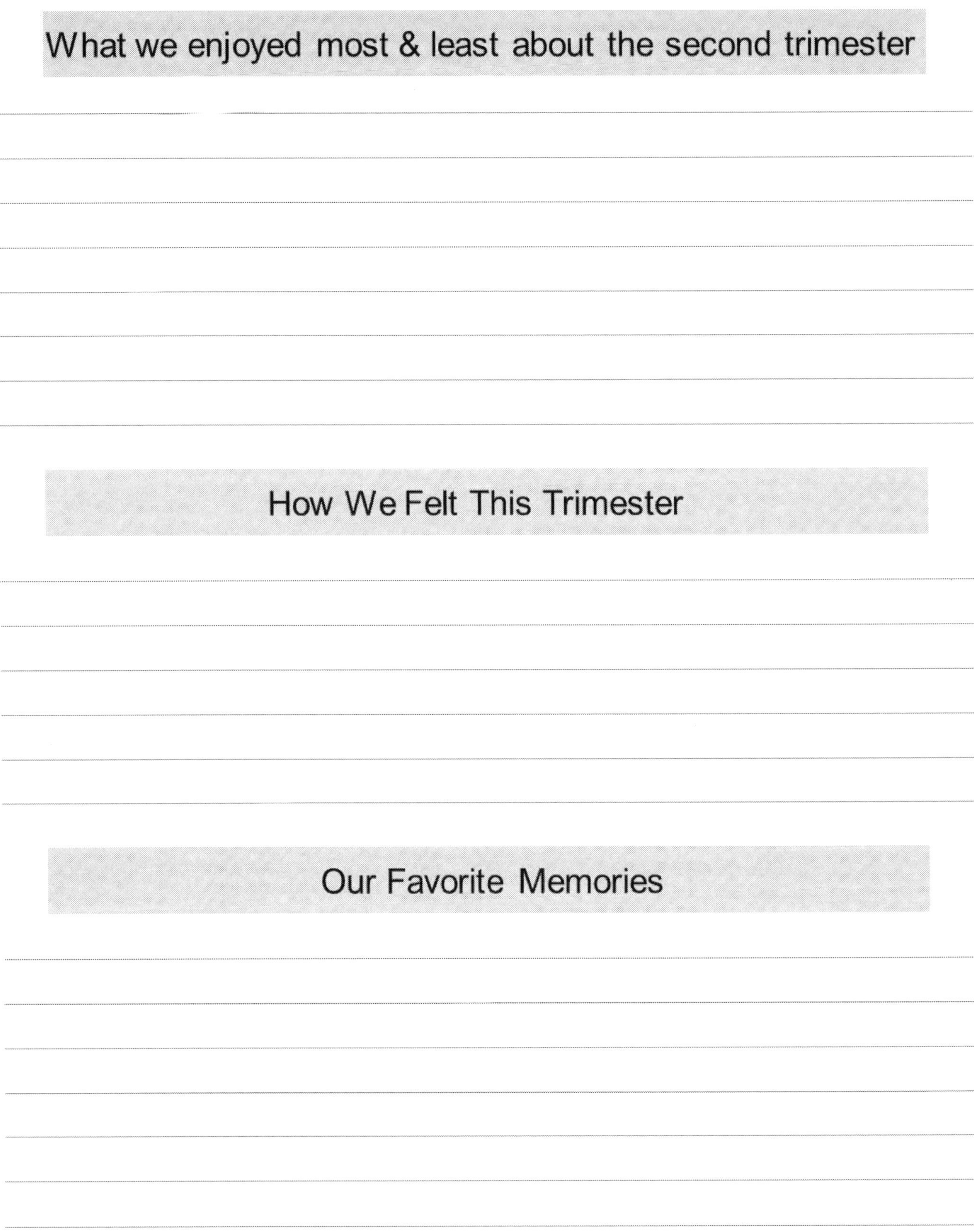

What we enjoyed most & least about the second trimester

How We Felt This Trimester

Our Favorite Memories

Our Pregnancy Journal Week 29

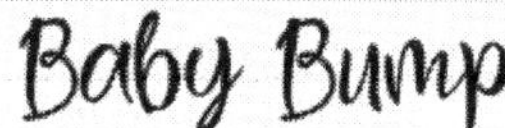

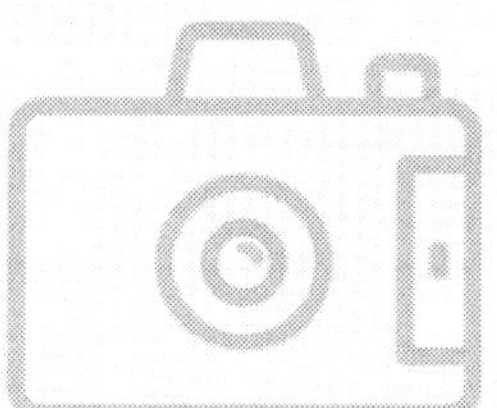

My Weight:

Belly Circumference:

Baby in Progress....Fun Facts

* Baby is the size of a big butternut squash, 15" long, & 2.5 lb.
* Baby's brain continues to develop the neurons needed for intelligence & personality.
* Baby's muscles get stronger, and a combination of this strength and less room in the womb, makes baby's kicks feel stronger.

What we want to remember most about this week:

Our Pregnancy Journal Week 30

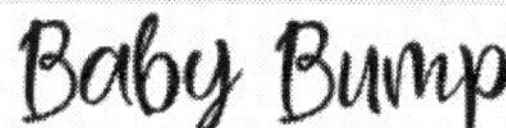

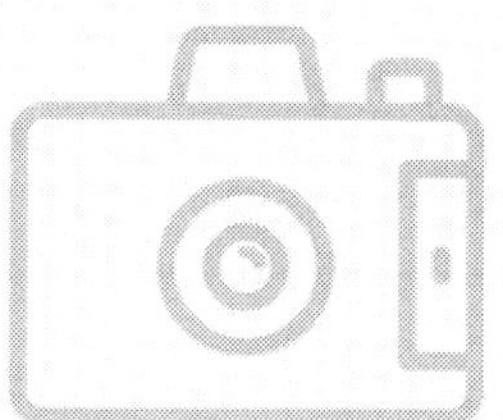

My Weight:

Belly Circumference:

Baby in Progress....Fun Facts

* Baby is the size of a big cabbage, weighs 3 lb, & is 15 ¾" long.
* As the baby continues to grow, the belly is quickly expanding too.
* If you haven't yet tried shining a flashlight on the belly, don't forget to do so as you may get a response (kick) from baby.

What we want to remember most about this week:

Our Pregnancy Journal

Week 31

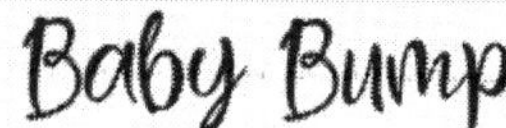

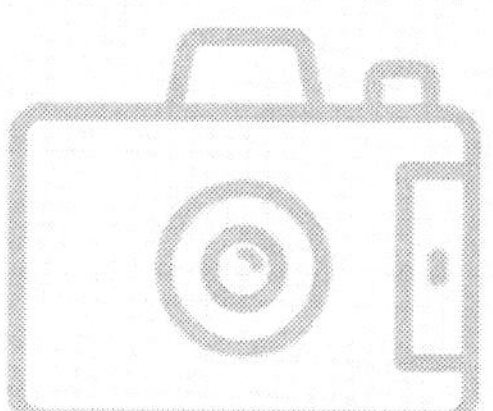

My Weight:

Belly Circumference:

Baby in Progress....Fun Facts

* Baby is the weight of a coconut, about 31/3 lbs.
* Baby is getting longer & bigger, so he/she takes on the curled-up, fetal position in utero until birth now.
* Braxton-Hicks contractions may be noticed now, in preparation for the eventual birth.
* The mom is putting on about a pound a week now as the baby fattens up and grows before birth.

What we want to remember most about this week:

Our Pregnancy Journal

Week 32

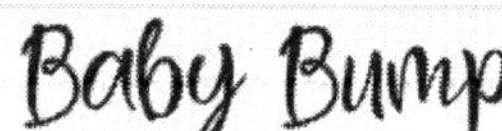

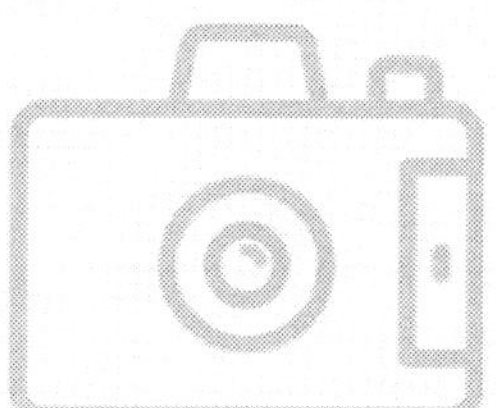

My Weight:

Belly Circumference:

Baby in Progress....Fun Facts

* Baby is 16 ¾" long, & weighs approx. 3 ¾ lb.
* If born now, baby has a good chance of surviving & being healthy, although baby's lungs aren't fully developed yet.
* Fine hair on the baby (lanugo) begins falling off. Of course, the hair on the head, eyebrows, and eyelashes remain.

What we want to remember most about this week:

Our Pregnancy Journal

Week 33

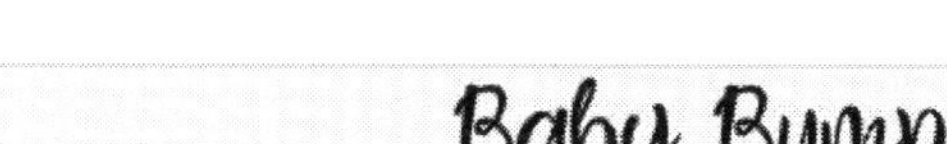

Baby Bump

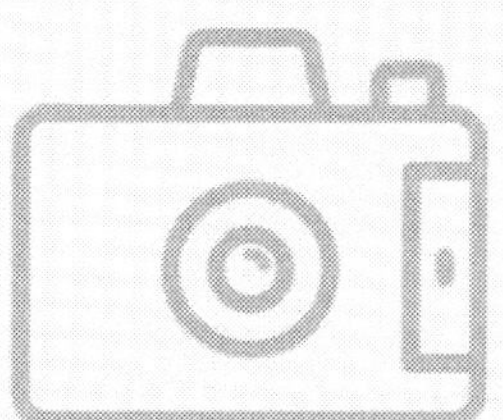

My Weight:

Belly Circumference:

Baby in Progress....Fun Facts

* Baby is the weight of a pineapple, weighs 4 lb, & is 17" long.
* You may notice that your baby's activity level & responses are dependent on your own actions, such as whether you've just eaten or you're in a noisy environment.

What we want to remember most about this week:

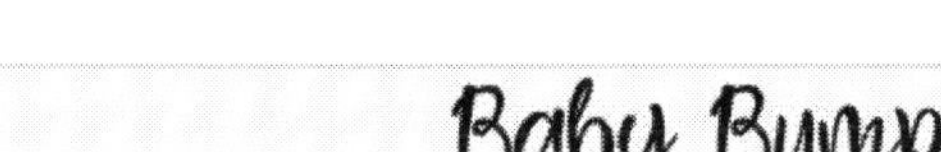

Week 34

Baby Bump

My Weight:

Belly Circumference:

Baby in Progress....Fun Facts

* Baby is 18" long, & 4 ¾ lb, and roughly the size of a cantaloupe.
* All the bones are fully developed now, except for the ones on the skull that remain soft, required for passage through the birth canal.
* Baby's organ systems are almost all ready to work on their own.

What we want to remember most about this week:

Our Pregnancy Journal

Week 35

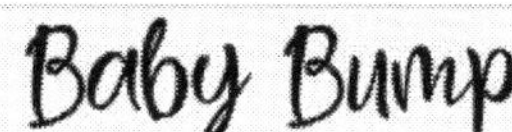

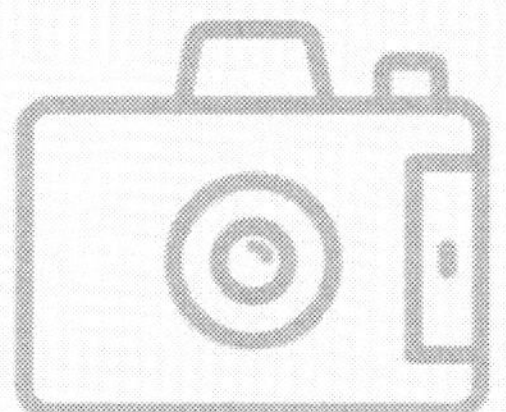

My Weight:

Belly Circumference:

Baby in Progress....Fun Facts

* Baby is the weight of a large honeydew melon at 5 ¼ lb. and is approx. 18" long.
* The amniotic fluid surrounding baby is decreasing. 97% of babies are head-down and "drop" down into the pelvis around this time, in preparation for the birth.
* Expect baby to increase by ½ pound per week now.

What we want to remember most about this week:

Our Pregnancy Journal Week 36

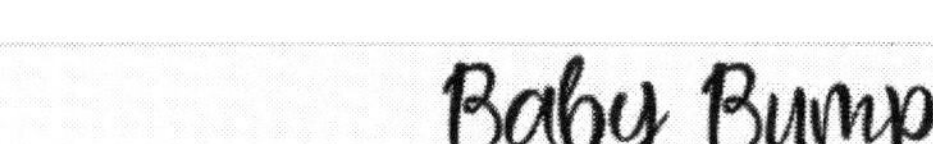

Baby Bump

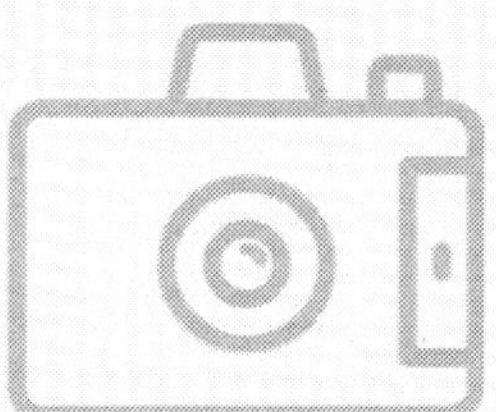

My Weight:

Belly Circumference:

Baby in Progress....Fun Facts

* Baby is 18.5" long, & weighs close to 6 lb.
* The waxy white coating (vernix caseosa) on baby is mostly now gone.
* Baby's born now have an excellent survival rate, but most ideal is a few more weeks in the womb to increase weight and fat depositions for thermoregulation.

What we want to remember most about this week:

Our Pregnancy Journal

Week 37

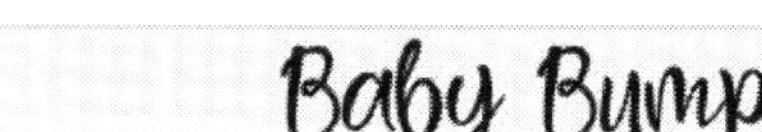

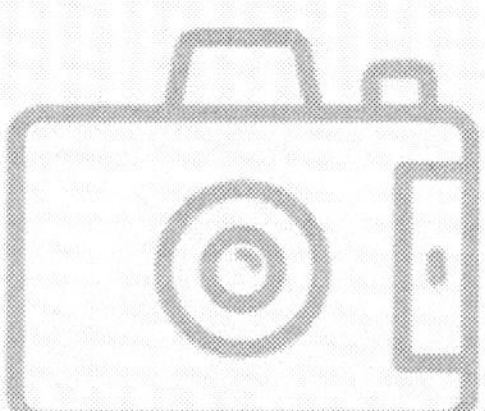

My Weight:

Belly Circumference:

Baby in Progress....Fun Facts

* Baby is approximately 19" long, & 6.5 lb.
* Baby is considered full-term if born now.
* Antibodies are passed to baby through the umbilical cord.

Baby's grasp is improving, ready to grasp your fingers (and hearts) when born.

What we want to remember most about this week:

Our Pregnancy Journal

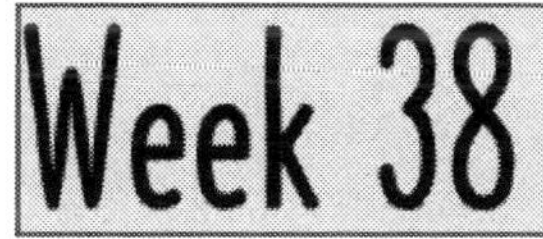

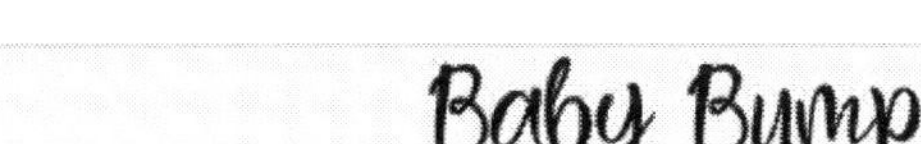

Baby Bump

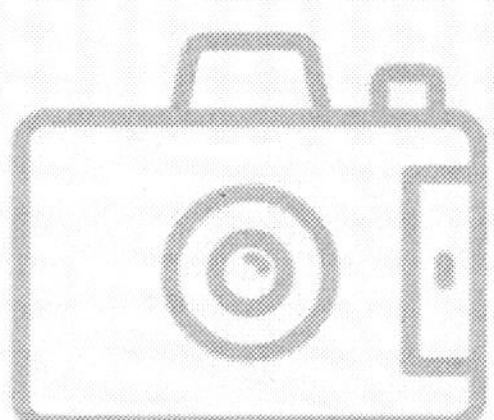

My Weight:

Belly Circumference:

Baby in Progress....Fun Facts

* Baby weighs about 7 lb, & is 19.5" long.
* Baby continues to improve his/her breathing, circulation, & digestion.
* Baby's reflexes such as rooting for the nipple and sucking are present.

What we want to remember most about this week:

Our Pregnancy Journal Week 39

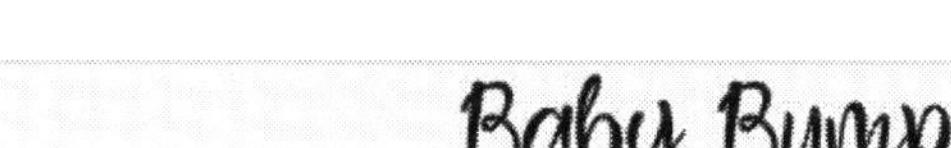

Baby Bump

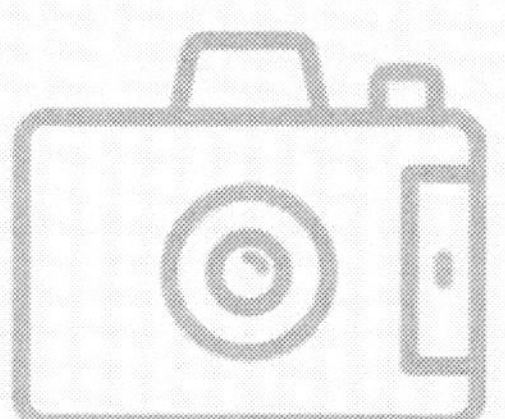

My Weight:

Belly Circumference:

Baby in Progress....Fun Facts

* Baby is approximately the weight of a watermelon, around 7 1/4 lb., and 20" in length.
* If you haven't given birth yet, baby is ready to meet his/her mommies any day now!

What we want to remember most about this week:

Our Pregnancy Journal

Week 40

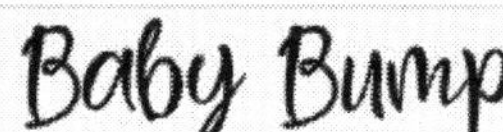

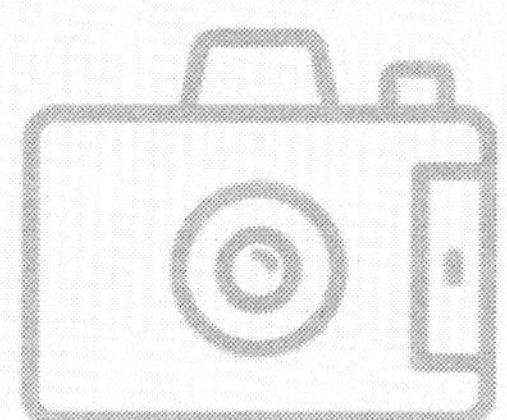

My Weight:

Belly Circumference:

Baby in Progress....Fun Facts

* Baby is the size of a pumpkin, weighs approx. 7.5 lb, & a bit over 20" long. But keep in mind that babies come in different weights and heights, so this is approximate!
* Baby is coming soon! But if baby doesn't come this week, don't worry. Only 5% of babies are born on their actual due dates.
* If you haven't yet packed your overnight hospital bag, you don't want to delay this any longer.

What we want to remember most about this week:

Our Pregnancy Journal

Week 41

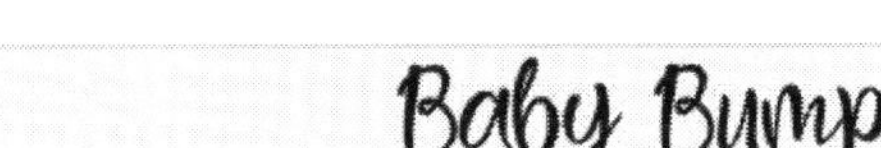

Baby Bump

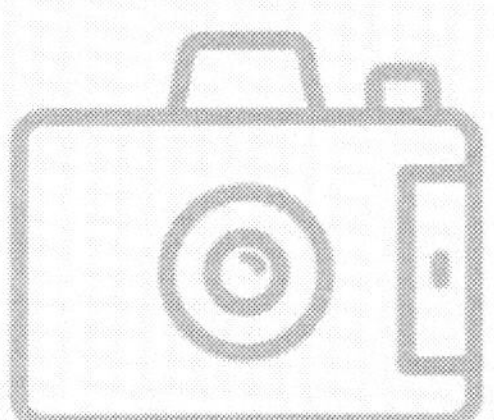

My Weight:

Belly Circumference:

Baby in Progress....Fun Facts

* It should be any time now! Enjoy the last few days of the pregnancy. You'll miss feeling the baby's movements in your womb after birth.

What we want to remember most about this week:

Our Third Trimester

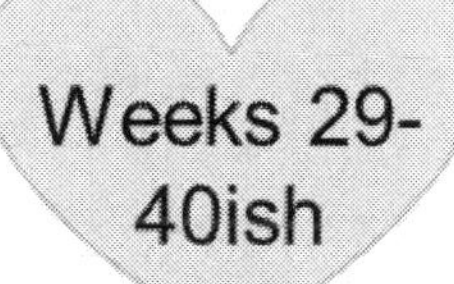

What we enjoyed most & least about the third trimester

How We Felt This Trimester

Our Favorite Memories

Fun Predictions

______________'s Prediction

Boy/Girl:

Date of birth:

Birth weight:

Time of birth:

Hours in labor:

Hair color:

______________'s Prediction

Boy/Girl:

Date of birth:

Birth weight:

Time of birth:

Hours in labor:

Hair color:

______________'s Prediction

Boy/Girl:

Date of birth:

Birth weight:

Time of birth:

Hours in labor:

Hair color:

______________'s Prediction

Boy/Girl:

Date of birth:

Birth weight:

Time of birth:

Hours in labor:

Hair color:

Fun Predictions

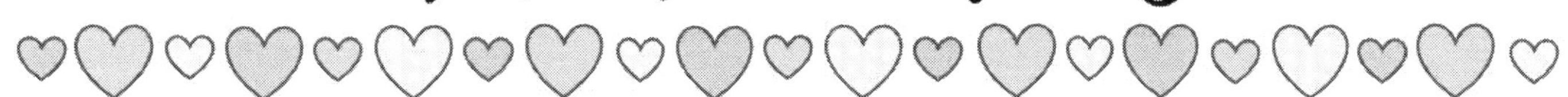

______________'s Prediction

Boy/Girl:

Date of birth:

Birth weight:

Time of birth:

Hours in labor:

Hair color:

______________'s Prediction

Boy/Girl:

Date of birth:

Birth weight:

Time of birth:

Hours in labor:

Hair color:

______________'s Prediction

Boy/Girl:

Date of birth:

Birth weight:

Time of birth:

Hours in labor:

Hair color:

______________'s Prediction

Boy/Girl:

Date of birth:

Birth weight:

Time of birth:

Hours in labor:

Hair color:

Newborn Baby Shopping Checklist

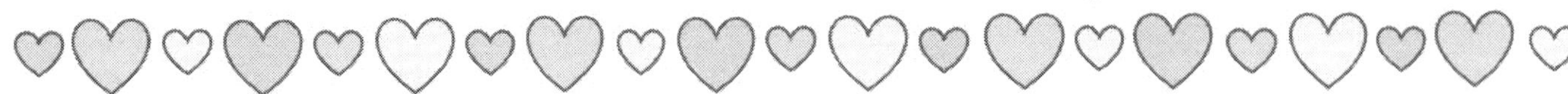

TIP: Keep in mind that baby grows quickly so don't buy too many clothes or diapers of the same size before baby is born. Don't forget to sign up for prenatal classes and Baby CPR classes.

Clothing

- [ ] Onesies
- [ ] Sleepwear
- [ ] Undershirts
- [ ] Socks
- [ ] Slippers
- [ ] Pants or shorts
- [ ] Shirts
- [ ] Dresses
- [ ] Scratch prevention mittens
- [ ] Baby hat
- [ ] Sweaters and jackets for babies born in cool weather
- [ ] Snowsuit & mitts for baby born in winter

Sleeping

- [ ] Crib & mattress
- [ ] Sheets for crib
- [ ] Baby monitor
- [ ] Swaddling blankets
- [ ] Baby sling
- [ ]
- [ ]

Bathing

- [ ] Baby wash cloths
- [ ] Baby hooded towels
- [ ] Soft-bristled baby brush
- [ ] Baby body wash/shampoo
- [ ] Baby lotion
- [ ] Baby bathtub
- [ ]
- [ ]
- [ ]

Diapering

- [ ] Diaper rash ointment
- [ ] Diaper pad &/or change table
- [ ] Baby wipes
- [ ] Diapers
- [ ] Diaper pail
- [ ] Diaper bag
- [ ]
- [ ]
- [ ]
- [ ]
- [ ]

Feeding

- [ ] Formula
- [ ] Baby bottles, bottle liners, bottle brush
- [ ] Nipple cream
- [ ] Breast pump & milk storage bags
- [ ] Nursing pillow
- [ ] Burp cloths & receiving blankets
- [ ] Nursing bras & pads
- [ ] Bibs
- [ ] High chair

Miscellaneous

- [ ] Baby laundry detergent
- [ ] Infant car seat
- [ ] Stroller
- [ ] Baby thermometer
- [ ] Mobile for crib
- [ ] Rocking chair
- [ ] Night light
- [ ] Nasal bulb syringe
- [ ] Nail scissors
- [ ] Pacifiers
- [ ] Baby swing

Foods/Drinks to Avoid on Shopping List

FISH, MEATS, & EGGS

Avoid raw, undercooked or smoked meat, chicken, fish and shellfish, including sushi, oysters, and clams. Deli meats should be limited, & only eaten when cooked to kill potential bacteria. Liver and other organ meats are high in Vitamin A – consult with a dietician or your doctor before consuming too much during pregnancy. Also limit how often you eat tuna, salmon, & swordfish (higher mercury content). Avoid raw eggs & foods that contain them (raw cookie/cake batter, eggnog, etc.).

DAIRY

Avoid unpasteurised milk (be sure you drink pasteurised milk), soft cheeses such as blue cheese, feta, brie, and several other kinds of these soft cheeses. Be sure to research the kinds that are and aren't safe.

VEGGIES & FRUIT

Wash them all very well. Cook them, whenever possible. Raw sprouts (alfalfa, clover, radish, & bean sprouts) are a concern. Avoid bruised veggies & fruit, as bacteria may have invaded the damaged areas. Also avoid unripe papaya, which has similar effects to oxytocin, which stimulates labor.

MISCELLANEOUS

Speak to your doctor about which medications are safe/not safe. Be careful of herbal remedies – speak to your doctor first as many are unsafe during pregnancy. Avoid all alcohol & drugs. Avoid artificial sweeteners, limit caffeine intake, soda, and other fatty or high-calorie foods with no nutritional value. Avoid unpasteurised juices too. Avoid foods with excess salt and trans fats.

Disclaimer: This list does **not** include every food item you should avoid. It is up to you to do your research & speak to your healthcare provider if you're not sure.

Foods/Drinks to Add on Shopping List

SOME GOOD IDEAS

- A prenatal vitamin and mineral supplement is recommended. Ensure you are getting enough folate/folic acid for at least 3 months before and at the start of your pregnancy to reduce the risk of neural tube defects.
- Almonds and other mixed nuts
- Avocados
- Sweet potatoes
- Broccoli & dark leafy greens (well washed)
- Protein in lean, fully-cooked meats, poultry, turkey, veal, etc.
- Pasteurised milk
- Hard cheeses like cheddar
- Yogurt
- Cold-pressed olive oil
- Fully-cooked eggs and omelettes
- Oranges

RECIPE I'D LIKE TO TRY

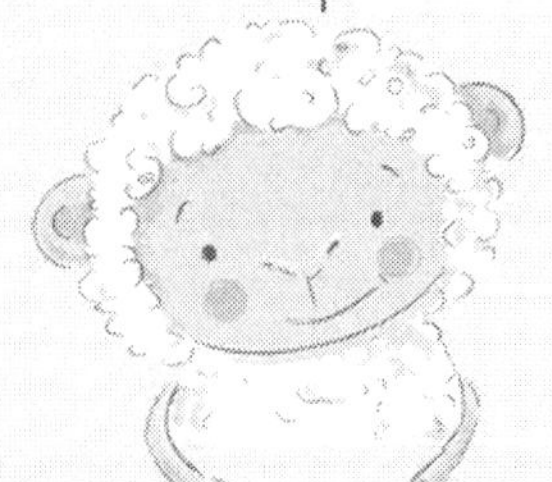

Disclaimer: This list does **not** include every food item you should be including in your diet. It is up to you to do your research & speak to your healthcare provider if you're not sure.

Growing a Healthy Baby Meal Planner

	Breakfast	Lunch	Supper	Snacks
Monday				
Tuesday				
Wednesday				
Thursday				
Friday				
Saturday				
Sunday				

Nursery Room Ideas

Favorite website examples:

Color scheme & theme ideas:

Draw out the layout, or add more notes:

Our Baby Shower

Friends & family who attended:

Games we played:

Baby Shower Photo:

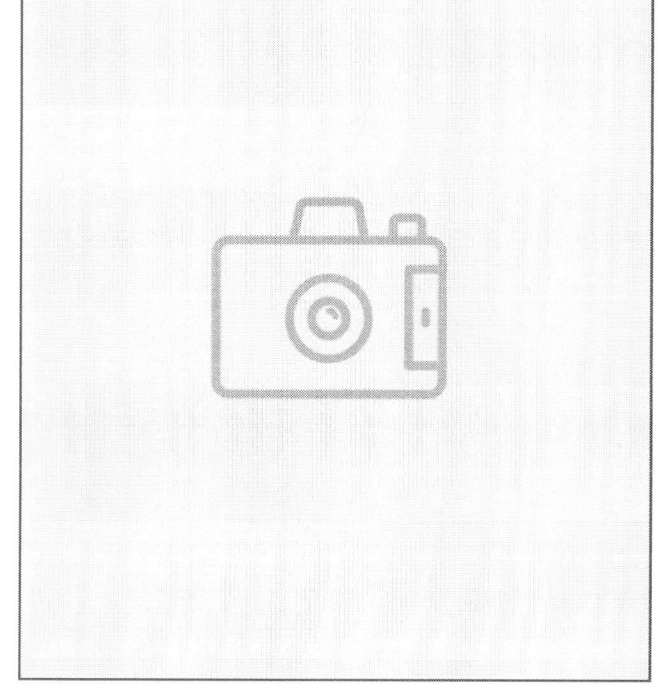

Our Favorite Memories of the Day:

Our Prenatal Appointments

Date: ______ Gestational Age: ______ My Weight Gain: ______ Blood Pressure: ______

Other important & memorable events (baby's heartbeat, what doctor said, etc.):

Date: ______ Gestational Age: ______ My Weight Gain: ______ Blood Pressure: ______

Other important & memorable events (baby's heartbeat, what doctor said, etc.):

Date: ______ Gestational Age: ______ My Weight Gain: ______ Blood Pressure: ______

Other important & memorable events (baby's heartbeat, what doctor said, etc.):

Date: ______ Gestational Age: ______ My Weight Gain: ______ Blood Pressure: ______

Other important & memorable events (baby's heartbeat, what doctor said, etc.):

Our Prenatal Appointments

Date: ______ Gestational Age: ______ My Weight Gain: ______ Blood Pressure: ______

Other important & memorable events (baby's heartbeat, what doctor said, etc.): ______

Date: ______ Gestational Age: ______ My Weight Gain: ______ Blood Pressure: ______

Other important & memorable events (baby's heartbeat, what doctor said, etc.): ______

Date: ______ Gestational Age: ______ My Weight Gain: ______ Blood Pressure: ______

Other important & memorable events (baby's heartbeat, what doctor said, etc.): ______

Date: ______ Gestational Age: ______ My Weight Gain: ______ Blood Pressure: ______

Other important & memorable events (baby's heartbeat, what doctor said, etc.): ______

Our Prenatal Appointments

Date: ____ Gestational Age: ____ My Weight Gain: ____ Blood Pressure: ____

Other important & memorable events (baby's heartbeat, what doctor said, etc.):

Date: ____ Gestational Age: ____ My Weight Gain: ____ Blood Pressure: ____

Other important & memorable events (baby's heartbeat, what doctor said, etc.):

Date: ____ Gestational Age: ____ My Weight Gain: ____ Blood Pressure: ____

Other important & memorable events (baby's heartbeat, what doctor said, etc.):

Date: ____ Gestational Age: ____ My Weight Gain: ____ Blood Pressure: ____

Other important & memorable events (baby's heartbeat, what doctor said, etc.):

Our Prenatal Appointments

Date: ____________ Gestational Age: ____________ My Weight Gain: ____________ Blood Pressure: ____________

Other important & memorable events (baby's heartbeat, what doctor said, etc.): ____________

Date: ____________ Gestational Age: ____________ My Weight Gain: ____________ Blood Pressure: ____________

Other important & memorable events (baby's heartbeat, what doctor said, etc.): ____________

Date: ____________ Gestational Age: ____________ My Weight Gain: ____________ Blood Pressure: ____________

Other important & memorable events (baby's heartbeat, what doctor said, etc.): ____________

Date: ____________ Gestational Age: ____________ My Weight Gain: ____________ Blood Pressure: ____________

Other important & memorable events (baby's heartbeat, what doctor said, etc.): ____________

Our Sonogram Photos

Insert Sonogram Photos here and/OR describe what you saw/felt at the ultrasound(s) of your baby.

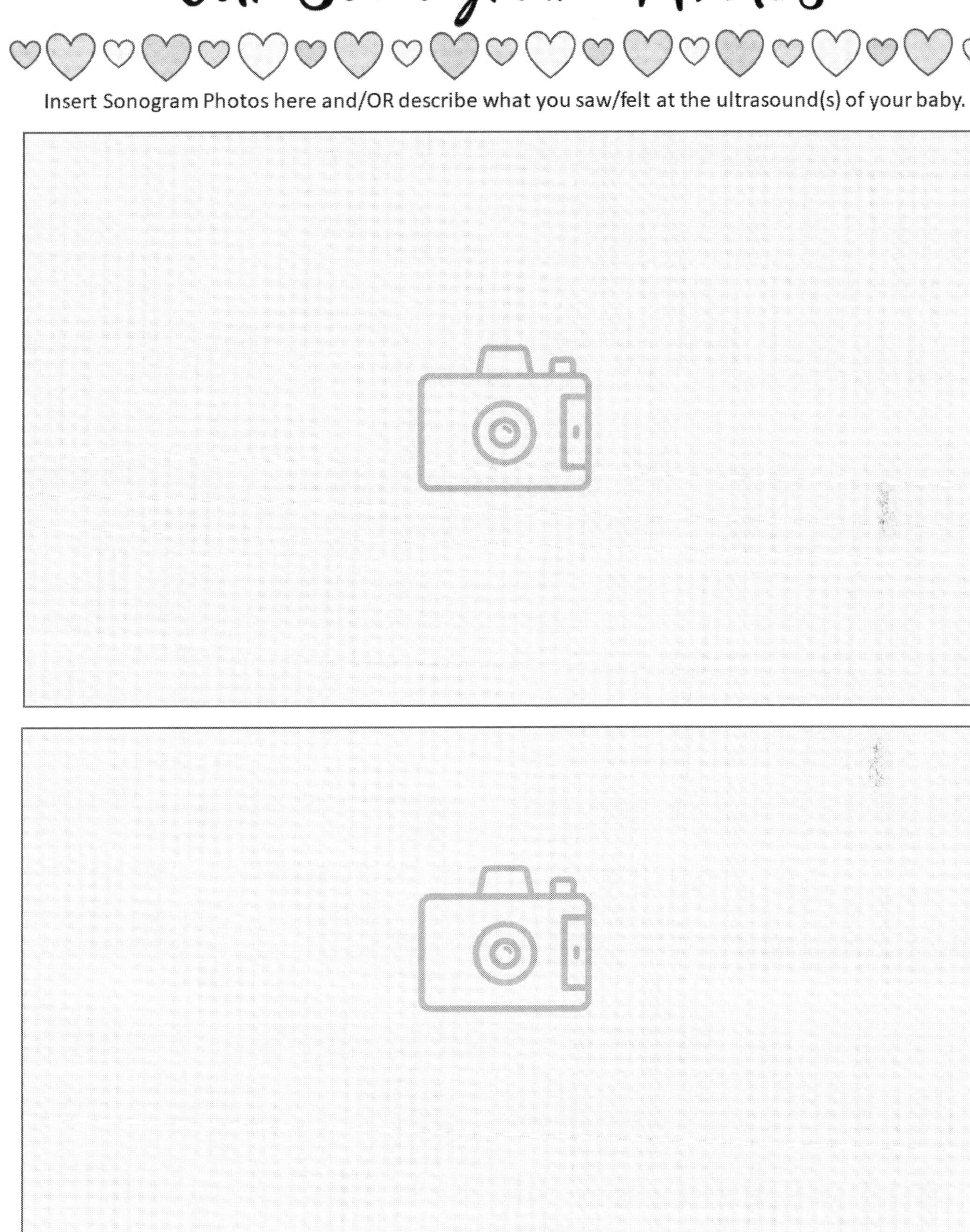

Fetal Movements Tracking Chart

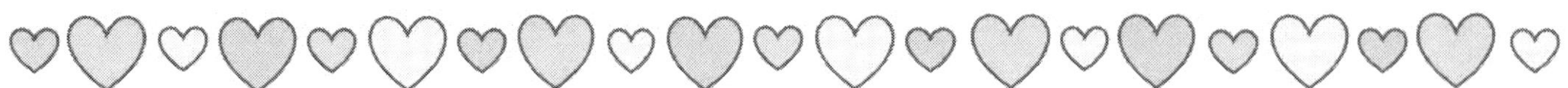

Date	Start Time	Baby's Movements						End Time
		✓	✓	✓	✓	✓	✓	

Date	Start Time	Baby's Movements						End Time
		✓	✓	✓	✓	✓	✓	

Important: Be sure to speak to your doctor or midwife to find out when and how to count your baby's movements.

Fetal Movements Tracking Chart

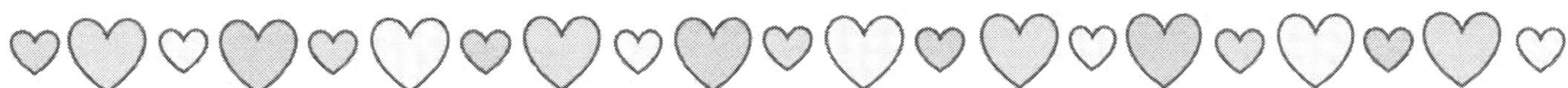

Date	Start Time	Baby's Movements						End Time
		✓	✓	✓	✓	✓	✓	

Date	Start Time	Baby's Movements						End Time
		✓	✓	✓	✓	✓	✓	

Important: Be sure to speak to your doctor or midwife to find out when and how to count your baby's movements.

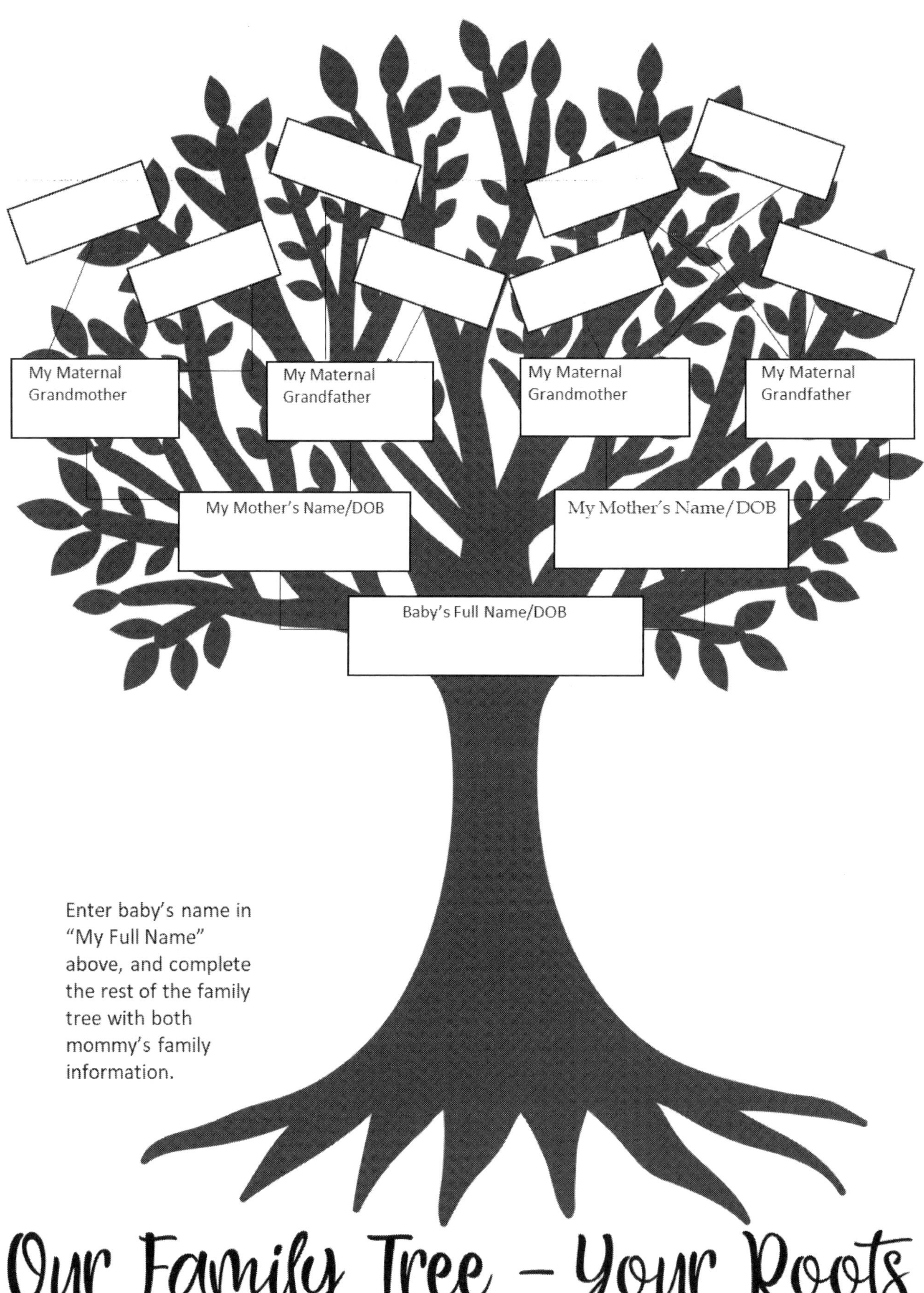

Enter baby's name in "My Full Name" above, and complete the rest of the family tree with both mommy's family information.

Our Family Tree – Your Roots

Create your own family tree from scratch if you need to represent divorces or deaths, and resulting remarriages that may have occurred in your families.

Baby's full name/DOB

Exercise During Pregnancy

Questions to ask our doctor or midwife & his/her responses:

(Keep in mind that some responses may vary depending on what trimester of pregnancy you're in and what is going on with you medically so be sure to revisit these questions with your doctor throughout your pregnancy)

Is it safe to exercise during my pregnancy?

Are there any risks of exercising while I'm pregnant?

What precautions should I take during exercise?

How much exercise should I get?

What are the best cardio and strength exercises I can do when I'm pregnant?

What exercises should I avoid during pregnancy?

What are warning signs that indicate I should stop exercising?

Names of Reputable Pregnancy & Exercise Websites:

Important Pre-Birth Questions

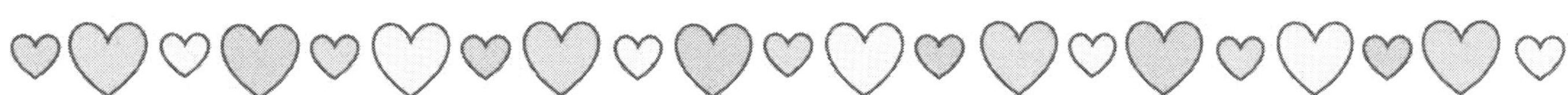

Do we want a midwife or obstetrician or our family doctor caring for me during the pregnancy, and why are we choosing one over the other?

What values are important to us when choosing our midwife or obstetrician (i.e. belief in natural process, breastfeeding knowledge, etc.)?

Is cord blood banking something we want to consider, and if so, where can we learn more?

If we have a boy, what are our thoughts on circumcision, and the risks and benefits?

Post more of our questions below:

Our Birth Plan

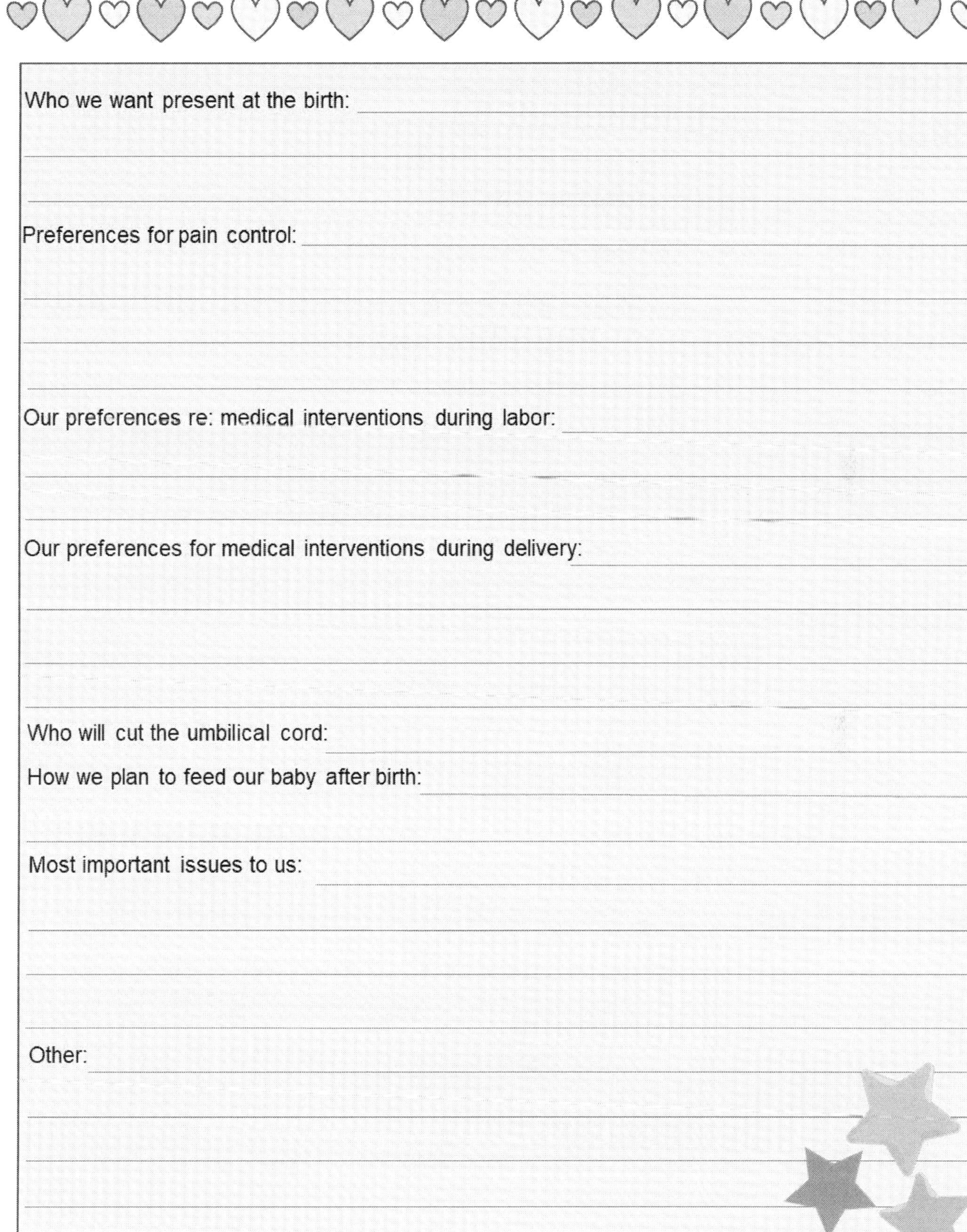
Who we want present at the birth:

Preferences for pain control:

Our preferences re: medical interventions during labor:

Our preferences for medical interventions during delivery:

Who will cut the umbilical cord:

How we plan to feed our baby after birth:

Most important issues to us:

Other:

Maternity Hospital Bag Checklist

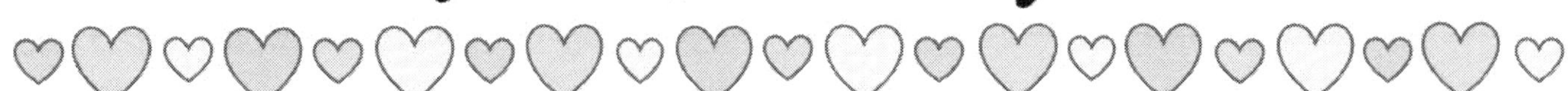

For Pregnant Mom

- [ ] Medical cards & insurance documents
- [ ] Birth plan
- [ ] Lip balm
- [ ] Maternity or loose-fitting pants & top
- [ ] Socks & Slippers
- [ ] Nightgown & robe
- [ ] Nursing pillow
- [ ] Massage oil or lotion
- [ ] Panties
- [ ] Nursing bras
- [ ] Nipple cream
- [ ] Toothbrush, toothpaste, & floss
- [ ] Hair brush
- [ ] Shampoo & conditioner
- [ ] Skin care & cosmetics
- [ ] Sheets for crib
- [ ] Deodorant/antiperspirants
- [ ] Glasses, contacts, solution
- [ ]
- [ ]
- [ ]

For Partner Mommy

- [ ] Snacks & water
- [ ] Phone, camera, video camera, & chargers
- [ ] Glasses & contact lens case
- [ ] Toothbrush & toothpaste
- [ ] Deodorant
- [ ] Change of clothes
- [ ] Book
- [ ] Money/credit card
- [ ]
- [ ]
- [ ]
- [ ]
- [ ]

For Baby

- [ ] Nightgown
- [ ] Sleepers
- [ ] Car seat
- [ ] Going-home outfit
- [ ] Socks & slippers
- [ ] Outerwear appropriate for the season
- [ ] Receiving blankets
- [ ] Pacifier
- [ ]
- [ ]
- [ ]
- [ ]
- [ ]

My First Love Letter to My Unborn Baby

My First Love Letter to My Unborn Baby

Our Baby Name Ideas

Mommy

Insert your name

Girl's Names

Boy's Names

Other thoughts:

** Each mom gets her own page, and then you can compare to see if you've chosen any of the same names. **

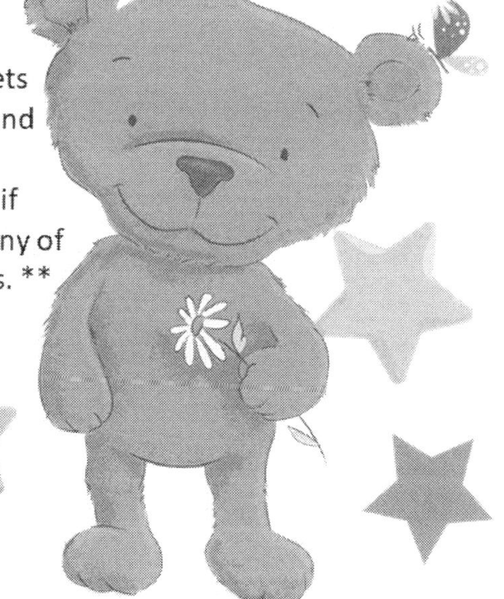

Our Baby Name Ideas

Mommy

Insert your name

Girl's Names

Boy's Names

Other thoughts:

** Each mom gets her own page, and then you can compare to see if you've chosen any of the same names. **

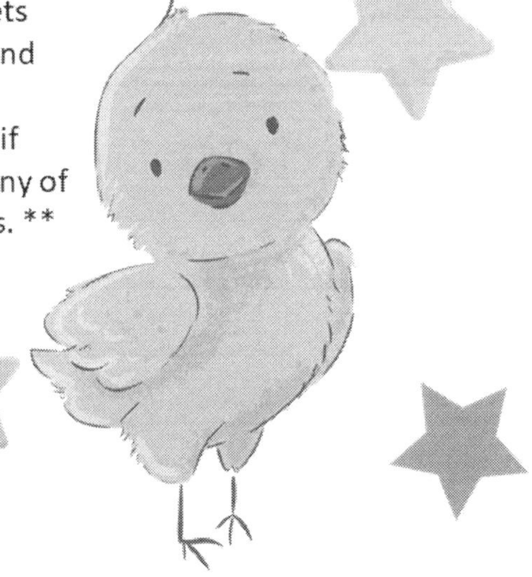

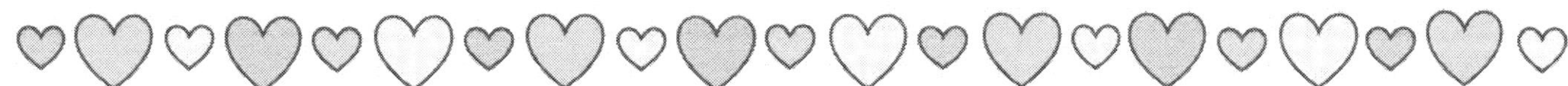

Our Pregnancy Photo Gallery

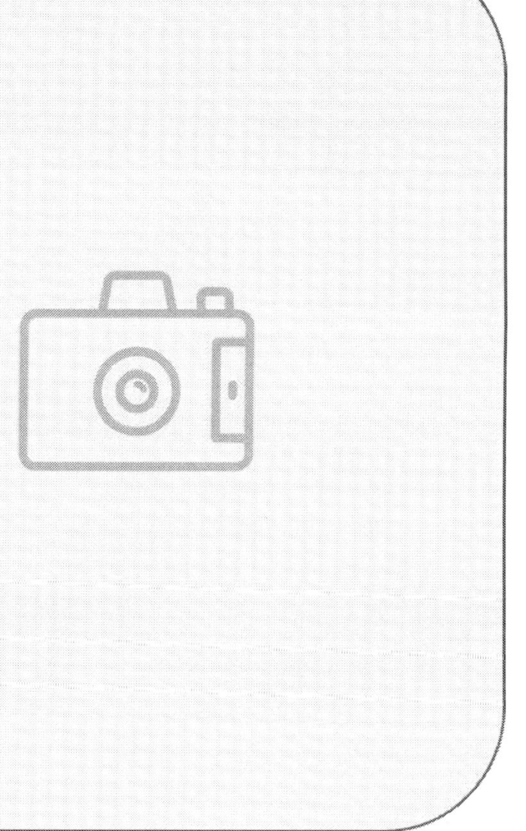

1st Month

Date of Photo:

2nd Month

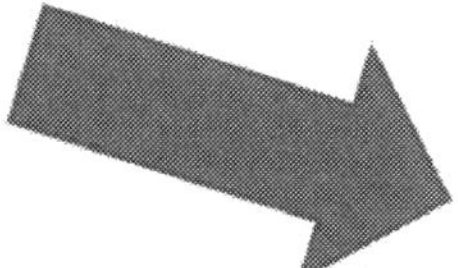

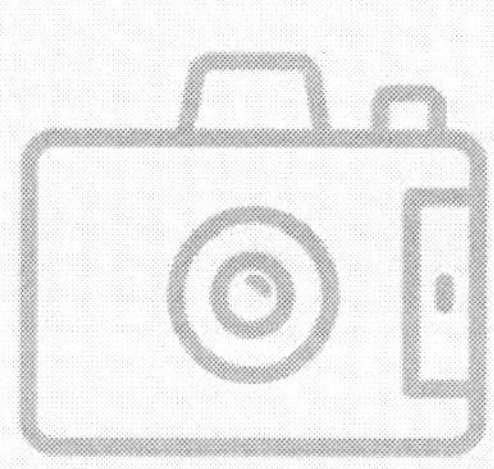

Date of Photo:

Use these pages if you prefer to add a monthly photo instead of weekly ones (or do both).

Note:

Although most people today leave their photos in a digital format in the cloud (or on their phones!), this is one time where you will want to print out and paste a monthly pregnancy photo to relive these precious memories easily in years to come.

In addition, to decrease the weight of the pages from the photos, the backside of the pages have purposely been left blank.

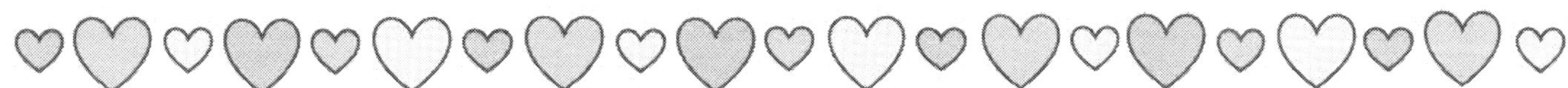

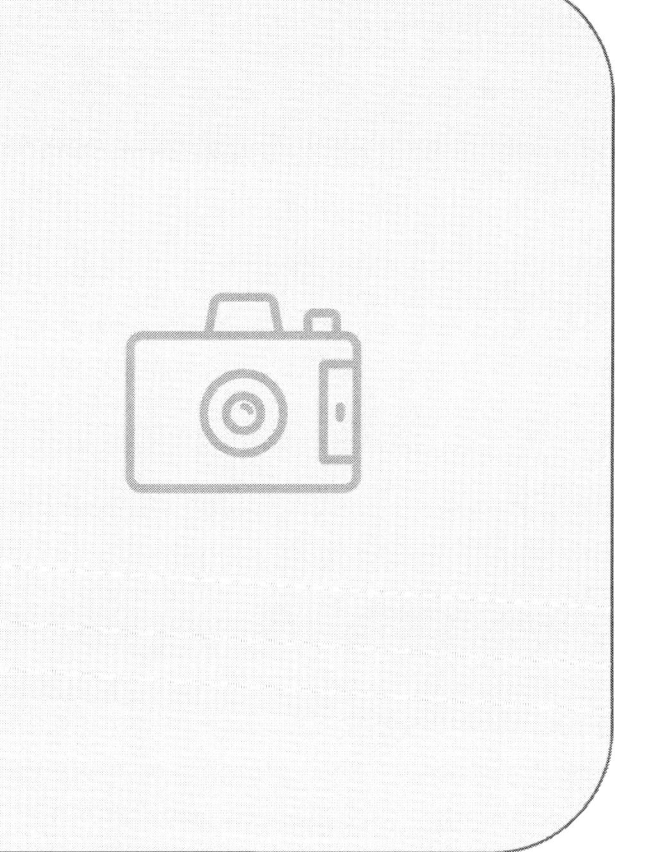

Our Pregnancy Photo Gallery

3rd Month

Date of Photo:

4th Month

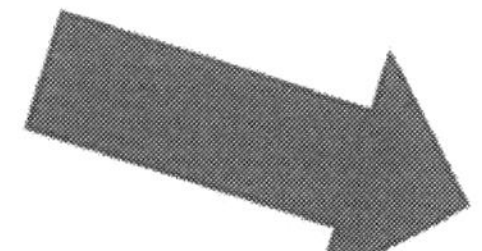

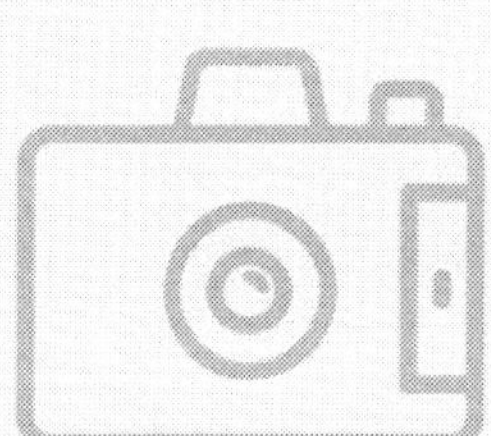

Date of Photo:

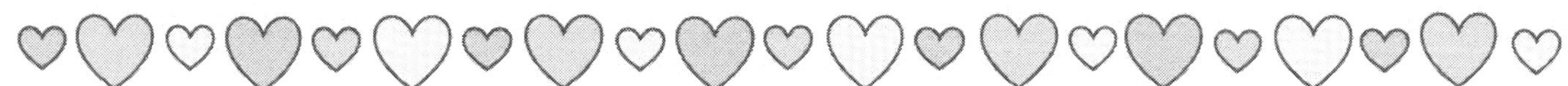

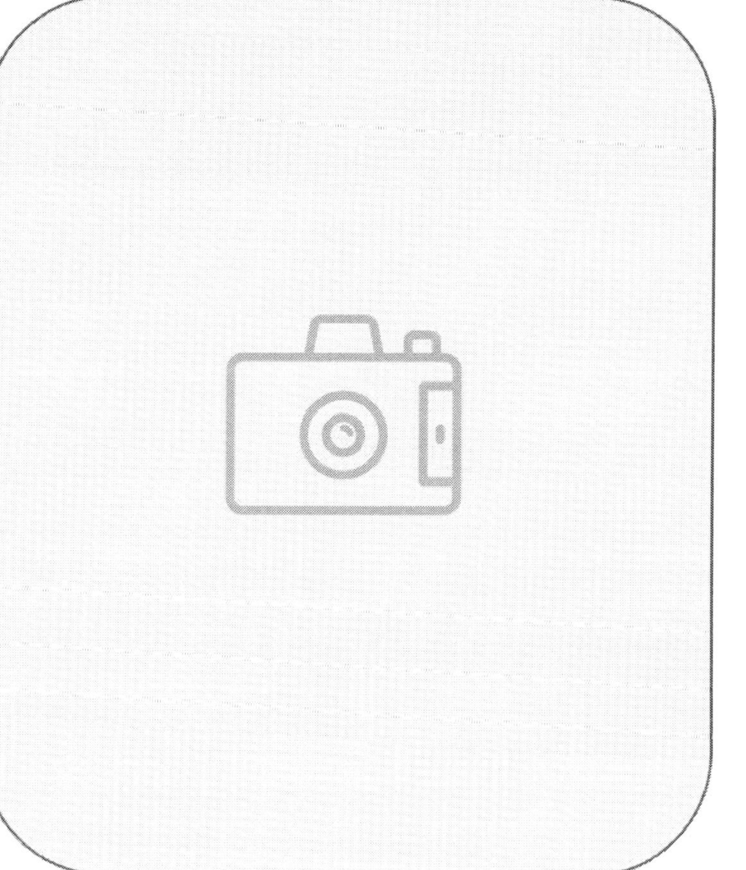

Our Pregnancy Photo Gallery

5th Month

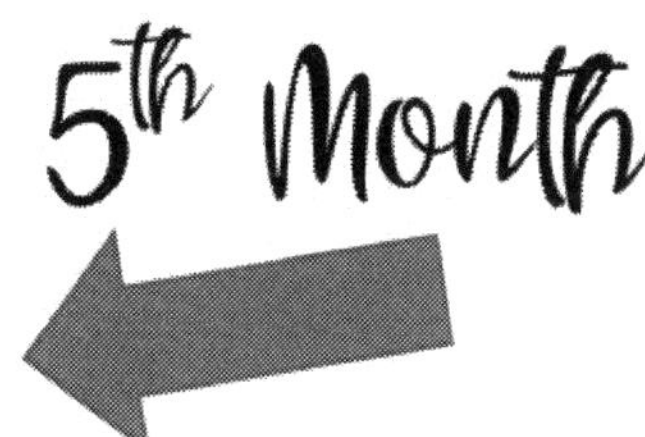

Date of Photo:

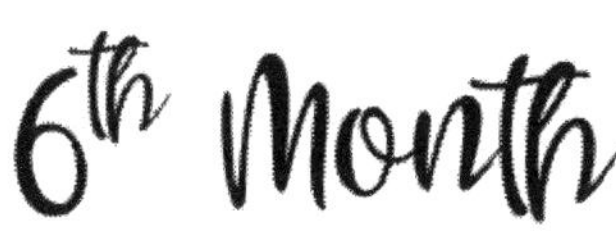

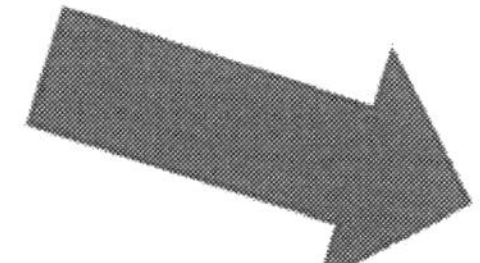

Date of Photo:

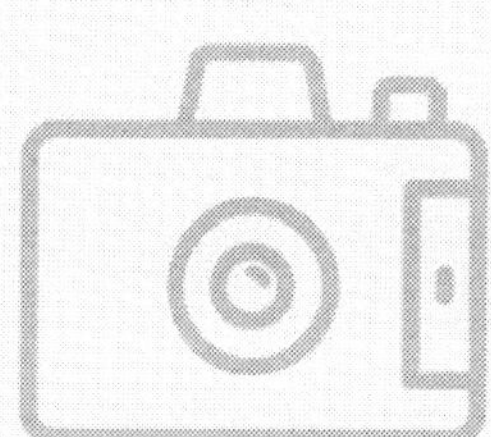

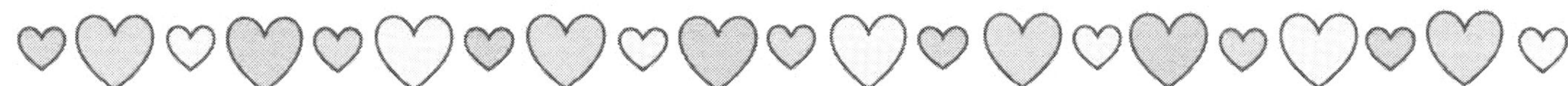

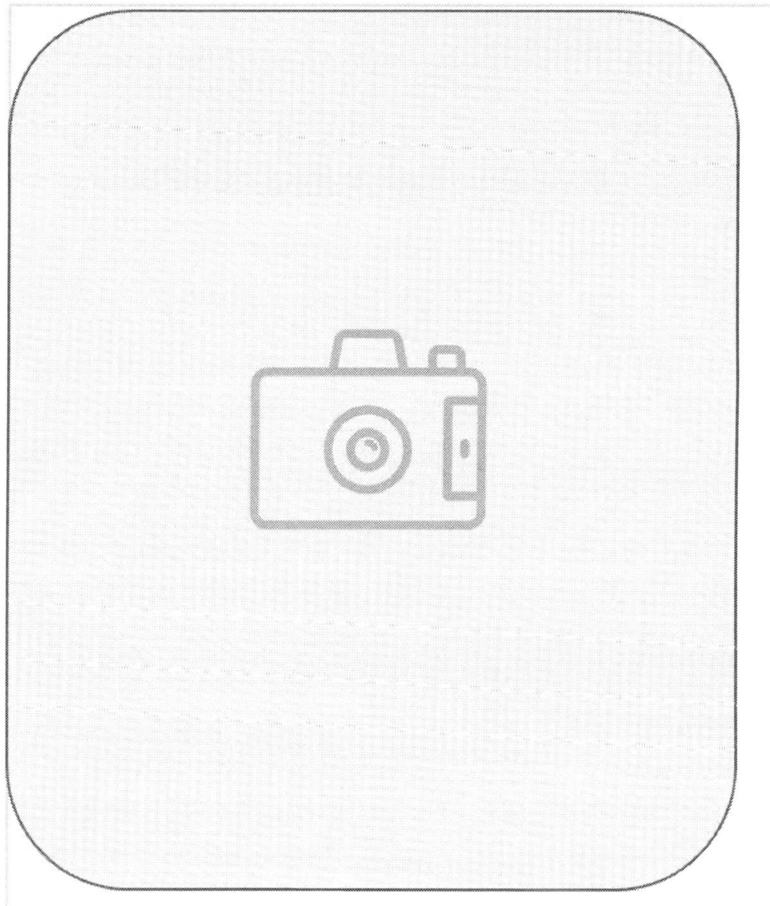

Our Pregnancy Photo Gallery

7th Month

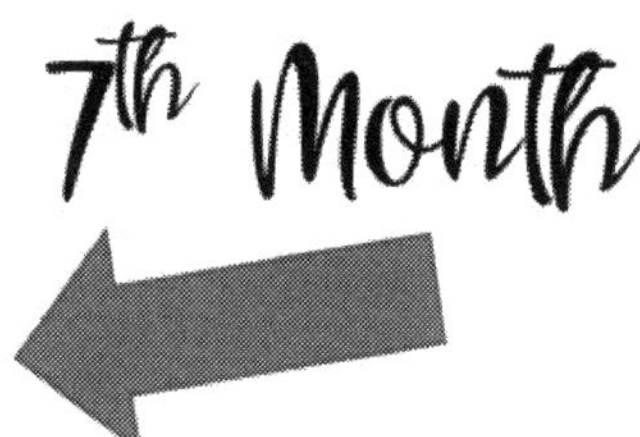

Date of Photo:

8th Month

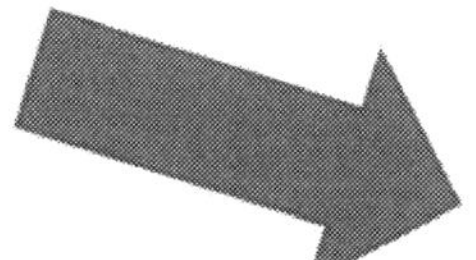

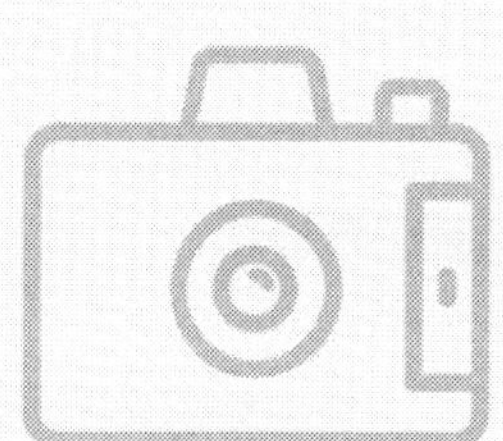

Date of Photo:

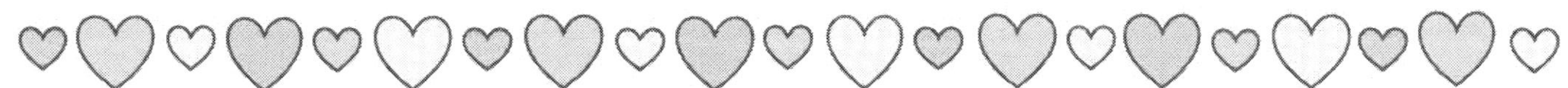

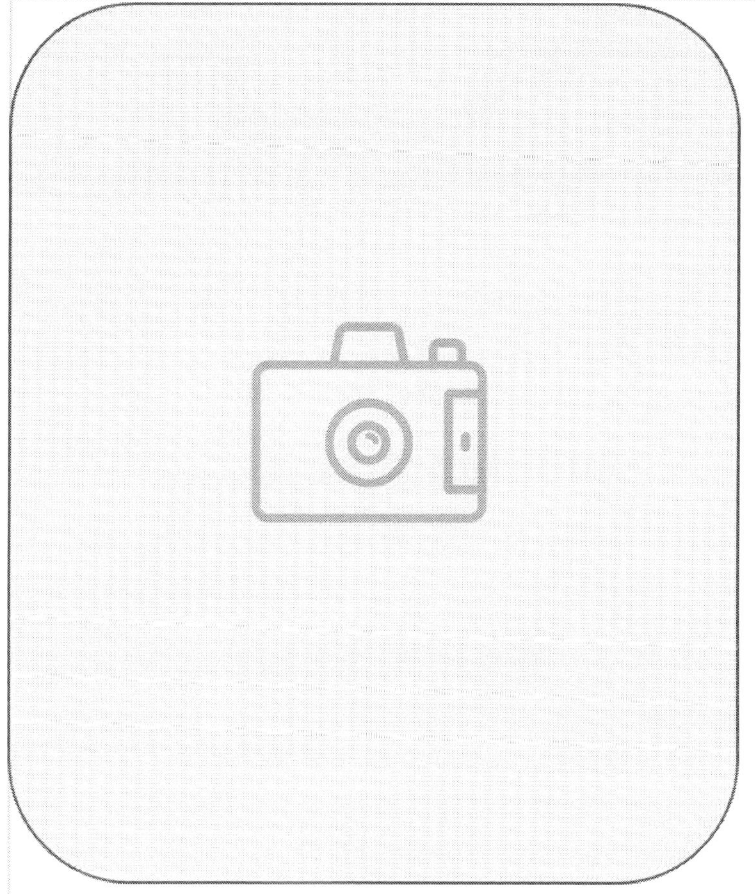

Our Pregnancy Photo Gallery

9th Month

Date of Photo:

Baby's 1st Photo

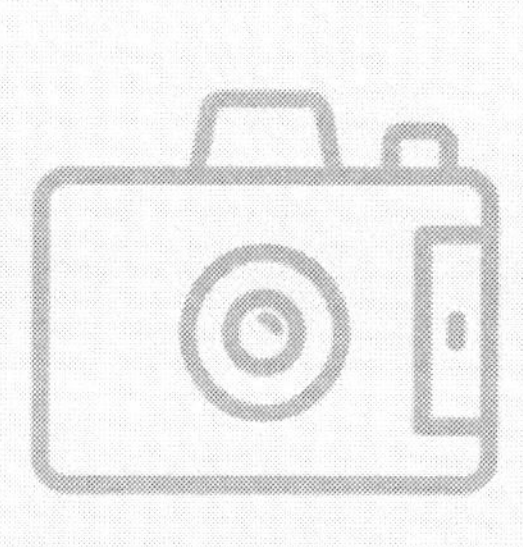

The Birth

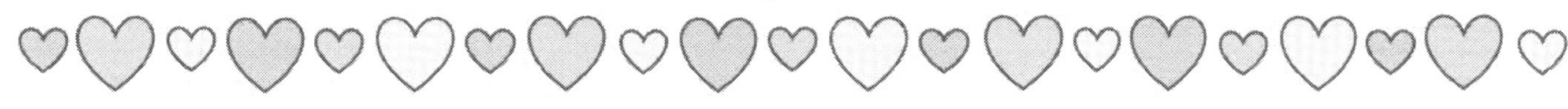

Baby's Full Name: ______________________________

WELCOME
TO THE WORLD!

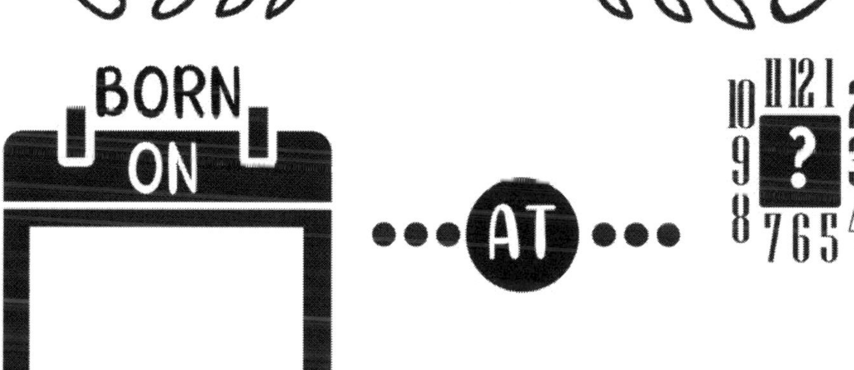

WEIGHING & MEASURING

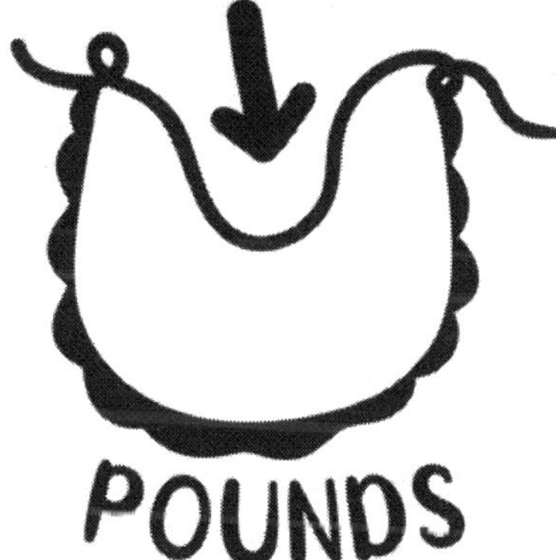

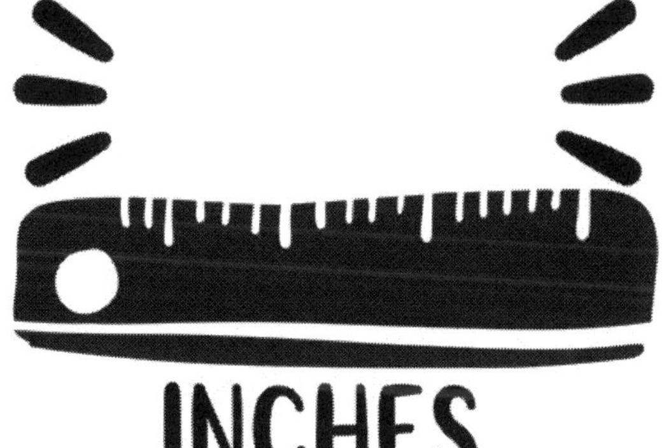

POUNDS

INCHES

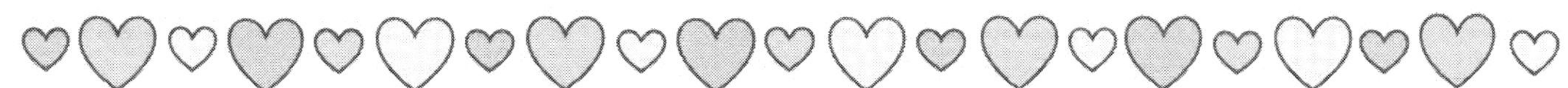

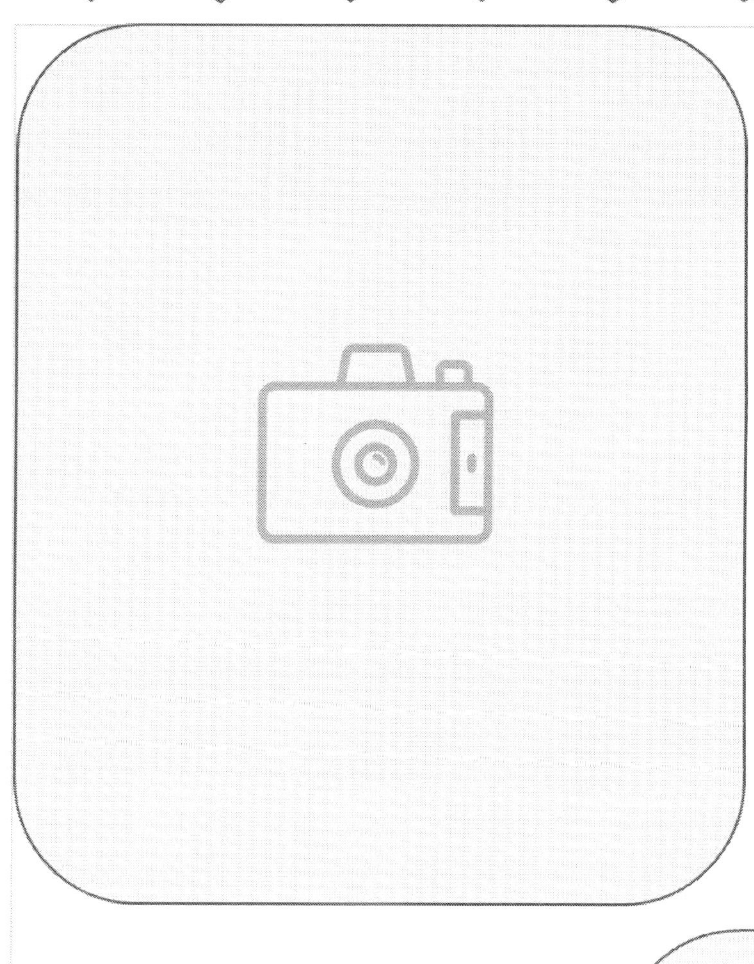

Our First Family Photos

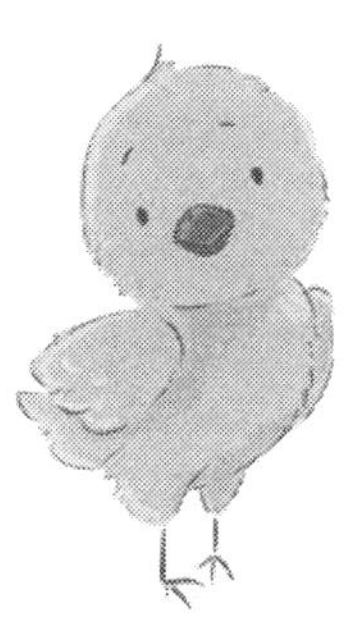

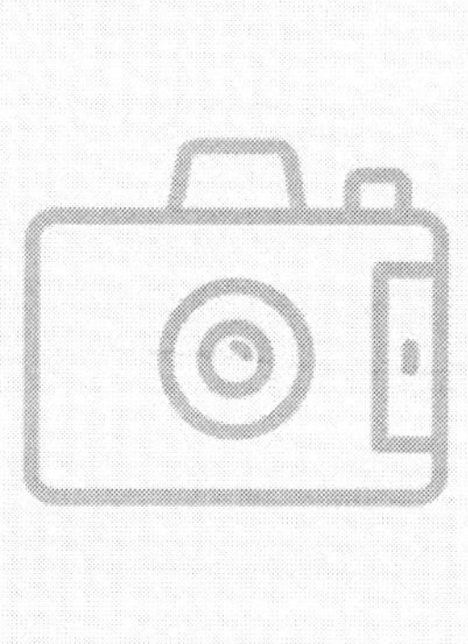

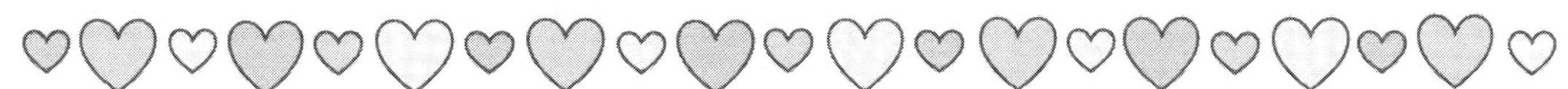

More of Baby's First Photos

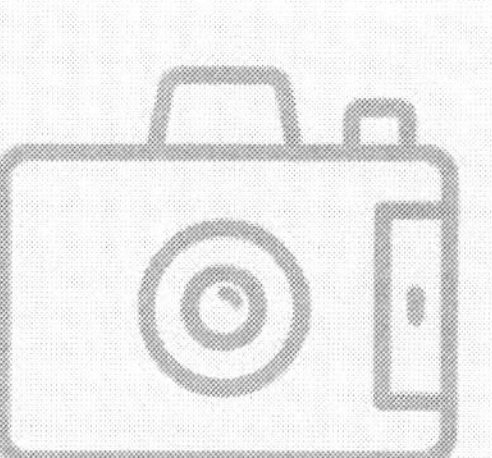

Trim photo to size and place here

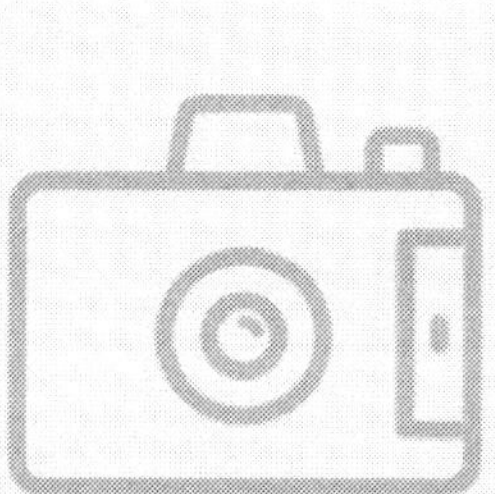

Trim photo to size and place here

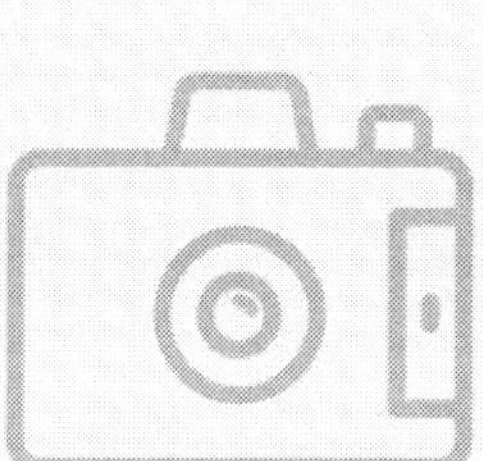

Made in the USA
Monee, IL
11 October 2023

47984316-c8d7-4b41-8b45-b7906a1b7a12R01